D0442961

THE

SECRETS

OF

PEOPLE

WHO

NEVER

GET SICK

THE
SECRETS
OF
PEOPLE
WHO
NEVER
GET SICK

GENE STONE

WORKMAN PUBLISHING · NEW YORK

Library of Congress Cataloging-in-
Publication Data is available.

ISBN 978-0-7611-5814-1

Cover design by Bob Perino
Author photo by Harold Levine
Design and Illustrations by E.Y. Lee

Workman books are available at special
discounts when purchased in bulk for
premiums and sales promotions as well
as for fund-raising or educational use.
Special editions or book excerpts can
also be created to specification. For
details, contact the Special Sales
Director at the address below or send an
e-mail to specialmarkets@workman.com.

WORKMAN PUBLISHING
COMPANY, INC.
225 Varick Street
New York, NY 10014-4381
www.workman.com

Printed in the United States of America
First Printing October 2010
10 9 8 7 6 5 4 3 2 1

This book is not intended as a substitute
for the medical advice of physicians.
Readers should regularly consult a
medical professional in all matters
relating to their health and particularly
with respect to any symptoms that may
require diagnosis or medical attention.

Grateful acknowledgment is made for permission
to reprint the following:

Page 17: "Pep-Up" recipe from Let's Eat Right to
Keep Fit, by Adelle Davis. Copyright © 1970 by
Adelle Davis. By permission of The Adelle Davis
Foundation.

Page 24: Tips on Calorie Restriction by
permission of the Calorie Restriction Society.

Page 25: Excerpts from How to Live to be
100—Or More, by George Burns. Copyright
© 1983 by George Burns, by permission of
George Burns's estate.

Page 30: "Chicken Soup" recipe from Cooking
Jewish, by Judy Bart Kancigor. Copyright © 1999,
2003, 2007 by Judy Bart Kancigor. Used by
permission of Workman Publishing Co., Inc.,
New York. All Rights Reserved.

Page 131: "Sweet Potato–Vegetable Lasagna"
recipe from The Engine 2 Diet by Rip Esselstyn.
Copyright © 2009 by Rip Esselstyn. By
permission of Grand Central Publishing.

Page 145: "Bug Crazy: Assessing the Benefits of
Probiotics," by Laura Johannes. Reprinted by
permission of The Wall Street Journal. Copyright
© 2009 Dow Jones & Company, Inc. All Rights
Reserved Worldwide. License number
2418860309904.

Page 178: Excerpts from Dr. Fulford's Touch of
Life, by Robert C. Fulford with Gene Stone.
Copyright © 1996 by Robert C. Fulford, DO, by
permission of Robert C. Fulford's estate.

The original material by Thomas Moore, Judith
Orloff, and Tim Sanders, and the advice of
Susan Smith Jones, were provided by those
authors. To learn more about each, please visit
their websites:
    Thomas Moore: Careofthesoul.net
    Judith Orloff: Drjudithorloff.com
    Tim Sanders: Timsanders.com
    Susan Smith Jones: susansmithjones.com

To all the people working toward
a health care system that pays as much
attention to the prevention of illness
as the curing of it.

Contents

INTRODUCTION IX

THE SECRETS

1. Blue Zones 3
2. Brewer's Yeast 10
3. Caloric Reduction 18
4. Chicken Soup 27
5. Cold Showers 34
6. Detoxification 39
7. Eating Dirt 48
8. Friends 55
9. Garlic 63
10. Germ Avoidance 70
11. Good Genes 79
12. Herbal Remedies 86
13. Hydrogen Peroxide 94

14. Lifting Weights 100
15. Napping 109
16. pH Balance 118
17. Plant-Based Diet 125
18. Positive Attitude 133
19. Probiotics 141
20. Running 149
21. Spirituality 157
22. Stresslessness 166
23. Stretching 173
24. Vitamin C 180
25. Yoga 188

AFTERWORD 195

ACKNOWLEDGMENTS 204

INDEX 206

Introduction

◆

Luigi Cornaro, a wealthy Venetian nobleman, was born into a prosperous family sometime around 1460. Like his peers in Renaissance Italy, Cornaro lived extravagantly, wearing imported, luxurious silk clothes, enjoying costly seats at popular jousts and parades, and eating whatever and whenever he wanted.

The life of an aristocrat consisted largely of the pursuit of pleasure: sport, intellectual exercise, and food. An average day might consist of waking to a generous breakfast, handling some business, downing a midmorning meal, then off to a horse race or a policy discussion with the doge (the Venetian chief magistrate). Then another meal and, after a nap, perhaps dancing and an extravagant supper.

Wealthy men like Cornaro typically consumed four or five massive meals a day. These feasts were opportunities to astonish guests with a lavishly spread table offering many courses and emphasizing difficult-to-obtain ingredients such as sugar (which was costly) and asparagus (which grew off-season only outside of Italy).

Here is an actual menu from a Venetian feast held during Cornaro's time.

◆

ROSEWATER-SCENTED WATER (FOR THE HANDS),
PASTRIES OF PINE NUTS AND SUGAR,
OTHER CAKES MADE WITH ALMONDS AND SUGAR
(SIMILAR TO MARZIPAN)

ASPARAGUS

TINY SAUSAGES AND MEATBALLS

ROAST GRAY PARTRIDGE WITH SAUCE

WHOLE CALVES' HEADS, GILDED AND SILVERED

CAPON AND PIGEON ACCOMPANIED BY SAUSAGES, HAM, AND WILD BOAR,
PLUS POTAGES (A TYPE OF THICK SOUP)

WHOLE ROAST SHEEP WITH SOUR-CHERRY SAUCE

A GREAT VARIETY OF ROAST BIRDS—TURTLEDOVE, PARTRIDGE, PHEASANT,
QUAIL, FIGPECKER—ACCOMPANIED BY AN OLIVE CONDIMENT

CHICKEN WITH SUGAR AND ROSEWATER

WHOLE ROAST SUCKLING PIG WITH AN ACCOMPANYING BROTH

ROAST PEACOCK WITH VARIOUS ACCOMPANIMENTS

A SWEETENED, SAGE-FLAVORED CUSTARD

QUINCES COOKED WITH SUGAR, CINNAMON, PINE NUTS, AND ARTICHOKES

VARIOUS PRESERVES MADE WITH SUGAR AND HONEY

TEN DIFFERENT TORTES AND AN ABUNDANCE OF CANDIED SPICES

◆

Menu from Mario Bendiscioli and Adriano Gallia, *Documenti di Storia Medievale, 400–1492* (Milan: Musia, 1970), *pp.* 267–68.

In the 1490s, as Cornaro approached his fortieth birthday (about ten years before an Italian aristocrat in the fifteenth century would have expected to die), he fell ill. His doctors informed him that if he wanted to survive, he'd have to moderate his diet. Most who received similar prescriptions ignored them, but not Cornaro. Having lived intemperately during the first part of his life, he was determined to live sensibly during the second part.

At the time, knowledge of the connection between diet and health was murky, so, as an experiment, Cornaro designed himself a new diet, cutting back drastically on the quantity of food he consumed. Each day, he limited himself to twelve ounces of solid food and fourteen ounces of wine (the water of its day, medieval wine was much lighter than today's vintages).

Cornaro's plan worked almost immediately. His health improved so dramatically that he continued his plan until age 68, when his doctors, worried that his food intake was too meager, insisted he eat and drink more generously. He complied but soon developed a mild fever, prompting him to return to a lighter menu, which he maintained for the rest of his life—till the age of 102.

Cornaro wrote about this plan in his four-volume book, often translated as *Discourses on a Temperate Life,* in which he articulated his philosophy that people should eat less as they grow older. He also elaborated on his belief that the body prefers rest to digestive action during periods of weakness, meaning that it is healthier to avoid food than to gorge on it. "There is no doubt," he wrote, "that if one so advised were to act accordingly, he would avoid all sickness in the future, because a well-regulated life removes the cause of disease."

Cornaro not only lived a very long time, but also remained healthy until just before his death. As he noted, "A long life full of disease and misery is worse than no life at all."

For centuries afterward, Cornaro's book was read and discussed by many other great writers and thinkers, including essayist Joseph Addison, Sir William Temple (Jonathan Swift's employer), and philosopher Francis

Bacon. But over the centuries, the book's influence waned, and today few people have even heard of Cornaro. However, his secret—calorie reduction—has resurfaced as a twenty-first-century approach to achieving health and longevity (see page 18).

Many other modern health secrets also originated long ago, only to lose favor or see their efficacy challenged by scientists looking for hard proof. But like Cornaro's, these secrets often have a surprising degree of validity.

For example, if you're prone to seizures, someone might have told you to be wary of the full moon, a warning medicine didn't take seriously until the 1990s, when researchers at Greece's University of Patras Medical School reviewed the records of 859 patients admitted for seizures and found "significant clustering of seizures" around the full moon.

You might also have dismissed the often-heard belief that fish is brain food as an old wives' tale—but many recent studies show that certain oils found in fatty fish (such as mackerel and sardines) play a significant role in brain development and functioning. Fish intake has also been associated with a slower rate of cognitive decline in aging patients, along with many other benefits.

For centuries, conventional wisdom held that cranberry juice will cure a bladder infection. Researchers at Harvard Medical School recently confirmed that cranberry juice actually does destroy bacteria clinging to the walls of the bladder. Similarly, an apple a day may well keep the doctor away; data from Ireland's University of Ulster suggest that high levels of certain chemical compounds found in apples help destroy colon-cancer cells. Moreover, Cornell University researchers have found that apples can prevent mammary cancers in animals.

Speaking of animals, it's often been said that having a pet is good for human health and well-being. New evidence corroborates the concept: Dog owners, for instance, tend to have fewer illnesses than their canine-free counterparts. "The simple act of petting an animal has been shown to lower blood pressure by inducing an instant relaxation response," says

Alan Beck, ScD, director of the Center for the Human-Animal Bond at
the Purdue University School of Veterinary Medicine.

For thousands of years, doctors used leeches as a bloodletting device;
the practice was only discontinued toward the end of the nineteenth
century. Recent medical research, however, indicates that leeches can
help cure many conditions, including osteoarthritis. Bee stings, too, have
made a comeback as a treatment to alleviate the symptoms of multiple
sclerosis. And if you have bedsores, one of the best remedies is the same
one that would have been prescribed for you in the year 1250. That
would be maggots, which devour dead tissue from open wounds and
eradicate bacteria by excreting a solution similar to ammonia.

In the Middle Ages, wealthy patients often drank suspensions of
finely ground gold (*aurum potabile,* or "drinkable gold") to ease the
symptoms of disease. The metal then fell out of favor for hundreds of
years, but at the end of the last century, studies revealed that small
quantities of liquid gold can strengthen the immune system and are
particularly useful in patients suffering from rheumatoid arthritis.
According to researchers from the Arthritis Research Centre of
Canada, "Gold therapy reduced the severity of arthritis in patients who
had a poor response with methotrexate, the standard drug used to
treat the disease."

———————◆———————

The popular remedies mentioned above aren't meant to suggest
that all notions held by mothers, midwives, scientists, or,
for that matter, anyone else are always accurate, or even useful.
Many are flawed. Some are foolhardy. Trepanation, the practice
of drilling holes in the skull to relieve the pressure that supposedly
caused all kinds of ailments, was practiced for more than five thousand
years throughout the world. It didn't work. For centuries many people
believed that coffee stunted growth; it doesn't. Copper bracelets,
supposedly beneficial for arthritis sufferers, do not appear to have any

benefit. The notion that staying outside in cold weather will give you a cold turns out to be wrong; the actual risk comes from staying inside in close contact with other people breathing germs on you.

The herb hemlock was once thought to be useful in reducing pain—but it also induced death. Cocaine was considered an excellent teeth whitener, as well as a treatment for morphine addiction; Sigmund Freud called it an excellent stimulant with no side effects or abuse potential.

There was a time when doctors routinely bled their patients; bloodletting was supposed to restore the balance of fluids in the body. When George Washington was ill, his doctors drained eighty ounces of blood from his body, likely precipitating his death.

In 1899, the respected *Merck Manual* recommended arsenic as a treatment for baldness. These days, the cancer-causing metal is listed as a toxic substance by the U.S. Environmental Protection Agency. The *Merck Manual* also listed coffee as a means to relieve insomnia. Other beverages, particularly liqueurs (which were first formulated as cures for everything from parasites to impotence), were mistakenly ascribed medicinal powers. The herbal liqueur Benedictine D.O.M. (*Deo Optimo Maximo,* "To God most good, most great"), originally formulated in 1510 from twenty-seven herbs and spices, was designed to fight malaria around the Benedictine Abbey at Fécamp on the north coast of France. Other liqueurs once believed to have restorative powers include the Belgian elixir d'Anvers (for stomachaches), the Greek mastic (also for gastric relief), and the French vervein du Velay (for increasing libido).

The eighteenth and nineteenth centuries were rife with a particularly infamous category of potions known as patent medicines (or nostrums), trademarked concoctions of dubious and sometimes harmful effect. Popular in Europe and the United States, these over-the-counter products promised miraculous curative powers over everything from tuberculosis and venereal diseases to colic and cancer, as well as the perennial advertising-industry favorite, "female complaints."

In reality, many patent medicines were benign, alcohol-based solutions, but some contained dangerous opiates or stimulants such as morphine, opium, or cocaine. For example, the opium-based laudanum, praised by the medical community as an effective pain-killer, was the scourge of the underclass in Victorian England. And heroin was once marketed by Bayer as a cough suppressant.

One of the more harmless concoctions included "snake oil," a term first innocently coined by a man named Clark Stanley for a benign ointment he created to cure muscle aches—but which came to mean any fraudulent medicine. (Stanley gained fame for killing live rattlesnakes as part of his demonstration at the 1893 Chicago World's Fair.) Although you can no longer buy Stanley's Snake Oil, other potions once marketed as patent medicines are still available (minus the health claims): Coca-Cola, Dr Pepper, 7UP, Angostura Bitters, and tonic water.

Even some very recent remedies have missed the mark. A few decades ago, it was thought that lying on a tanning bed in winter might keep vitamin D levels high and prevent seasonal depression—until the journal *Lancet Oncology* published findings showing that the probability of cancer increased by 75 percent in people who used tanning beds before the age of thirty. Such research led the International Agency for Research on Cancer to reclassify tanning beds as "a definite carcinogen," alongside tobacco products, arsenic, and mustard gas.

———————◆———————

Which health secrets make sense and which don't? Who can benefit most? How can you make sure that you live a long and healthy life? How can you manage to avoid sick days at the office?

How do you just flat-out manage avoiding being sick at all?

This book is designed to answer these questions, because all of us could profit from knowing what keeps other people well and how to stay well ourselves.

I certainly felt my health could stand improvement. For the past two decades, I've written extensively about health as a journalist and ghostwriter. As someone who believes that responsible writing can require participation, I've experimented with nearly every tip, technique, and tonic I've covered. (The exception: electroconvulsive therapy. The doctors interviewed offered me a free session, but I declined.)

This commitment means I've probably been tested more than nearly any other relatively healthy human being. I've been through body scans, ECGs, EKGs, DEXA bone-density scans, DEXA body composition scans, IgG food antibody tests, and 2D and Doppler echocardiograms. I've had my blood tested for C-reactive protein, homocysteine, fibrinogen, insulin levels, lipoprotein A, and I've taken a glucose challenge. I've had urinary and serum-amino-acid nutritional profiles taken, along with myriad lipid profiles; my cholesterol levels have been charted so frequently that they look like a plot of the Dow Jones Industrial Average. I've been tested for every possible allergy (I'm mildly allergic to cats, certain pollens, and mold). I've had my muscles studied, my organs examined, and my brain waves synched via a contraption placed on my head (instead of generating alpha waves, my brain tuned in to a local radio station).

I've also sampled countless spa treatments, from Bindi Shirodhara to Ayurvedic herbal rejuvenation, and submitted myself to dozens of New Age modalities, including candling, rebirthing, crystal therapy, past-life regression, and polarity therapy. I've had feng shui experts rearrange my home for better energy flow and seasonal affective disorder experts install lighting to boost my mood. I've undergone acupuncture, biofeedback, hypnotherapy, bioenergetics, the Alexander technique, Rolfing, reiki, and reflexology.

Being fairly obedient, I've generally tried everything experts have recommended, from exercising the 1980s way (cardiovascular and strength training) to working out the twenty-first-century way (interval training). I've let doctors attach electrodes to my scalp in sleep labs and allowed pros at consciousness labs to investigate the inside of my brain. I've experimented with Freudian therapy, Jungian therapy, primal therapy, cognitive therapy, aromatherapy, and EMDR (eye movement desensitization and reprocessing). I've talked to psychics about my health, and to pet psychics about my pets' health. (One of the latter suggested my cat was whining at night to warn me that the stairs in our apartment were dangerous.)

Despite all this, I always got sick at least twice a year. At some point every winter, I came down with a blistering sore throat that turned into a lingering cold. Then, in either late spring or early fall, a different kind of cold took over, one that started with a mild tickle in the throat, moved to my chest, then settled in my nose, where it lingered like a lazy guest who won't get off the couch, resting there indolently for days.

It has recently occurred to me that I was taking the wrong medicine. Instead of relying solely on experts, my thoughts have turned to people who don't depend on medical professionals—or any type of expert, for that matter—but who manage to stay healthy nevertheless.

I've known many such people in my life. While I was enduring one cold after another, they were happily living under the cover of some personal secret that kept them healthy even as I twisted, writhed, and sneezed, in thrall to whatever germ, virus, or unidentified alien life form was sweeping through my being.

Not that all such secrets are worthwhile—as mentioned, some are downright wrong, while others are simply strange. What all the secrets in this book share is that they seem to work for the people who promote them—often better than the solutions proffered by science. Despite centuries of lifesaving advances in medicine and public health, medical professionals still can't tell us how to stay well. The common cold is just as common as it was eons ago, and sickness itself shows no sign of abating. So why not look for solutions to sickness among those for whom the common cold is uncommon?

This became my mission for the last few years: to find people who didn't get sick, to find out why they didn't get sick, and then to see if their secrets were valid for others.

For the most part, these people who "never get sick" actually may

THE HANDS OF DR. SEMMELWEIS

◆

Sometimes the best health wisdom stays a secret not because its advocate doesn't tell people, but because no one believes him, as in the case of Ignaz Semmelweis.

Hungarian by birth, Semmelweis became a doctor in the 1840s and went to work in the maternity department of a Vienna hospital. At the time, many women giving birth contracted puerperal fever, a now rare infectious disease that was once the most common cause of maternal mortality in Europe.

Oddly, fewer cases of puerperal fever occurred when babies were delivered by midwives at the mother's home than by doctors at a maternity clinic. Many possible reasons were proposed; none could be proven. Then Semmelweis, who was obsessed with the problem, realized that medical students and doctors often entered the maternity wards directly from dissecting rooms, where they had been touching corpses. He concluded that mortality rates would drop if doctors simply washed and disinfected their hands before their next surgery or delivery.

Nobody believed him. At the time, there was no reason to think that unclean hands could cause disease—germ theory hadn't yet been proposed, much less proven. Semmelweis was ridiculed, but he didn't relent, fighting unsuccessfully for hand washing, becoming increasingly bitter and angry until 1865, when his wife and others committed him to an asylum. There he died two weeks later, reportedly due to a beating by the staff.

Cleanliness in the maternity ward and operating room did not gain widespread support until the late 1800s, after scientists (especially French chemist and microbiologist Louis Pasteur) developed the germ theory of disease. Today, Semmelweis is considered a pioneer in health care.

catch a slight cold now and then or suffer an occasional ache and pain here or there. What they don't have are the colds, flus, and fevers so many of us get so often. They also rarely have any serious diseases. Although they may have inherited some kind of genetic condition that manifested at some point, they've energetically fought it off—or in a few cases, did come down with a major illness but adapted their secret to the situation and achieved a solid recovery. Overall, they are living long and healthy lives.

To find them, I talked to friends, placed ads, searched down Internet connections, looked up old book collaborators, located former school classmates, and chatted with health care professionals, journalists, and editors. Because I've been writing about health for a long time, I was lucky to have a large list of connections upon which to draw.

I've known a few of those profiled in this book for many years. Susan Rennau and I attended high school together. Then there's my sixth-grade teacher (whom I haven't seen since, well, sixth grade). I met others through my career as a ghostwriter. I've written books for Rip Esselstyn, Gail Evans, and Robert Fulford. In the end, I interviewed approximately one hundred people, all of whom offered diverse, sometimes bizarre, secrets to health. The secrets presented here are ones that seemed destined to remain interesting over time, had the firmest basis in scientific fact, and were endorsed intelligently and articulately by their proponents.

Some of those *not* selected included closing the lid to the toilet before flushing (although some evidence does support this practice), taking various vitamin and nutritional supplements (in some cases, swallowing more than twenty pills a day), consuming certain foods (including oranges, apples, and pomegranates or less common foods, such as sea beans, fiddleheads, cardoons, and longans), eating a strict raw-food diet (or an even stricter *vegan* raw-food diet), placing a humidifier in every room, changing the shower curtain regularly, meditating in an isolation tank, getting a flu shot, and bathing the cats or dogs frequently. All are possible secrets for health but are not as verifiable, interesting, and replicable as those chosen.

What follows are twenty-five of what I believe are the most worthwhile secrets to health. You, the reader, get the final say on which ones make the most sense for *you*.

THE
SECRETS

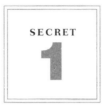

Blue Zones

RICARDO OSORNO FALLAS

Each day, twenty-eight-year-old Ricardo Osorno Fallas wakes up at 6:00 A.M. in Hojancha, a regional capital in the Nicoya Peninsula of northwestern Costa Rica. Like many Costa Ricans, Ricardo still lives at his parents' home (along with three brothers and sisters), where he'll probably stay until he marries

Breakfast is a bowl of oatmeal or some *gallo pinto,* the national dish of rice and beans, with corn tortillas. (Literally translated, *gallo pinto* means "mottled rooster," referring to the color the rice turns when fried with beans.) After eating, Ricardo rides his bike a couple of kilometers to his job as a liaison for a local ecotourism company that specializes in showing foreigners the rain-forest nature preserves around Hojancha.

He works until noon, then bikes back home for lunch, the largest meal of the day: rice, black beans, meat, and corn tortillas washed down with a glass of cold water. Dessert is a piece of locally sourced tropical fruit, such as an orange, pineapple, or banana.

After lunch, Ricardo heads back to his office, where he stays until 4:00 P.M. Upon returning home, he helps his mother or father around the house or pays a visit to his ninety-three-year-old grandmother. Then, after a light dinner, he practices with a group that performs traditional Nicoyan dances, such as the *arma de café,* as well as regional favorites like salsa and the merengue.

Before going to bed at midnight, Ricardo usually puts in a few hours of work on his master's thesis, a business plan for a marketing agency he hopes to start upon receiving his degree in marketing from the Hispano-American University of Costa Rica.

"We have a very relaxed pace of life here," he says. "We live with a sense of tranquility that is hard to find [elsewhere]—even in Costa Rica. The air that you breathe in Hojancha is just better than in any other place."

Ricardo is in excellent health, as is his entire family. In fact, they are up to three times as likely as the average American to reach the age

THE FIVE CONFIRMED BLUE ZONES

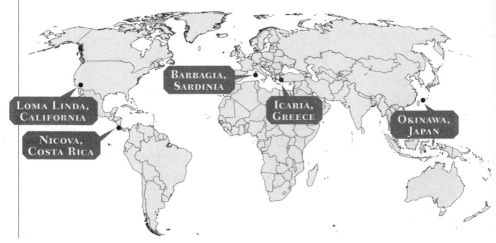

of one hundred. Their secret, however, isn't something that any of them invented or even thought about. The secret is that they live in the middle of a Blue Zone.

The Facts on Blue Zones

Blue Zones are geographic areas with high concentrations of the world's longest-lived people. The term was coined by journalist and explorer Dan Buettner, who, in partnership with longevity researchers, has spent the last decade traveling to the healthiest corners of the world to unearth the secrets of their inhabitants.

So far, five Blue Zones have been confirmed:

* In the rural, mountainous region of Barbagia, Sardinia, Italy, people are working as shepherds well into and past their seventies, and not infrequently becoming centenarians.

* The island of Okinawa, Japan, has the highest concentration of centenarians in the world, despite having weathered years of subjugation by invaders as well as widespread famine during and after World War II.

* Tucked into the polluted confines of greater Los Angeles, the city of Loma Linda is home to a community of nine thousand Seventh Day Adventists, currently the longest-living group of people in America.

* Icaria, Greece, has the highest percentage of ninety-year-olds on the planet, a cancer rate 20 percent lower than the rest of Greece, and almost no dementia.

* And then there's Nicoya, where Ricardo and his family live, a notable exception to the rule that people in developing countries have shorter life spans than those in developed ones.

To understand some of the reasons why Blue-Zoners live healthier, longer lives, let's take another look at Ricardo's daily routine.

First, his diet. Inhabitants of Blue Zones tend to have diets high in nutrients and low in calories and to avoid heavily processed foods. Each of the staples in Ricardo's diet (rice, beans, corn, and fruit) has a benefit. Rice is packed with vitamins, minerals, and antioxidants as well as being low in sodium. Beans contain potassium, magnesium, antioxidants, and fiber and are high in protein and carbohydrates but low in calories and fat. Corn is a cancer fighter as well as a valuable source of vitamin C. Moreover, the maize used in Ricardo's tortillas has been cooked in lime, causing it to undergo a process called nixtamalization. This process increases the corn's calcium content and improves the bioavailability of niacin and other vitamins already in the grain.

Furthermore, by snacking on fresh fruits, Ricardo avoids unnecessary fats and sugars while packing even more vitamins into his diet.

Ricardo washes down his food almost exclusively with water. Avoiding sugary soft drinks associated with heart disease and obesity is good in itself, but there is also something special about the water in Nicoya: It is very hard, meaning it contains minerals, including calcium and magnesium, associated with the reduction of cardiovascular disease.

Despite making no effort to limit the quantity of food he eats, Ricardo unknowingly consumes a calorie-restricted diet because his menu is high in protein but low in caloric density. He also limits his calorie intake by eating a light dinner early in the evening. Smaller meals are part of a practice, common in Blue Zones, that the Okinawans call *hara hachi bu*. Roughly translated, this means eating until you are 80 percent full; by eating until you are no longer hungry, as opposed to feeling full, you can, some doctors assert, eat 20 percent less—the difference between gaining weight and losing it.

Calorie restriction (see Secret 3, page 18) is currently the subject of intense study in the medical community, with a growing number of doctors acknowledging that it may ward off many of the diseases associated with aging.

Ricardo's next secret: His close ties to his family, which he calls "the solid base responsible for the moral and spiritual formation of Costa Ricans."

The concept of the family in Costa Rica, especially in rural areas, "revolves around togetherness and mutual support," he says. Families are the social nuclei of all Blue Zones, with a special emphasis placed on caring for the elderly. Numerous scientific studies have linked strong social networks to a host of benefits, including reduced obesity, post-operative pain, and risk of chronic illness. Social networks, which provide a sense of support and belonging, are especially important for older folks. They also play a role in creating what Costa Ricans call a *plan de vida,* or what the Okinawans call *ikigai:* a reason to live. A strong commitment to family, friends, community, and the environment give many Hojanchans a shared sense of purpose and keeps them busy and motivated far into their silver years. Again, science supports the concept: A 2009 study by the Rush Alzheimer's Disease Center in Chicago showed that staying busy and having a sense of purpose helps people live longer.

"DOCTOR, NO MEDICINE— *we are machines made to live, organized expressly for the purpose. Such is our nature. Do not counteract the living principle. Leave it at liberty to defend itself, and it will do better than your drugs."* —NAPOLÉON BONAPARTE, FRENCH EMPEROR

And according to Ricardo, a commitment to protecting the environment is a common sentiment among Nicoyans. "Everyone here grows up with a very environmentally conscious mentality," he says. "Although we want to use our natural resources, everything we do takes the environment into consideration."

Despite his active day, Ricardo considers Hojancha to be a very relaxed place compared with bigger Costa Rican cities like San José. Stress is a well-established killer, and by avoiding it while staying busy, Ricardo and other Blue-Zone dwellers help decrease their incidences of sickness and prolong their lives.

Equally important, physical activity is an integral part of Ricardo's daily routine. Because his family has never owned a car, he always walked or biked to and from school, including the return home for lunch. Now, with his daily bike rides and dancing hobby, he gets plenty of exercise without putting too much strain on his body.

Unfortunately, some benefits of Blue-Zone living can be obtained only from being born in and living in a Blue Zone. These areas all are home to strong and relatively isolated gene pools. Buettner, who has written about his findings in a book called *The Blue Zones,* estimates that our genes dictate about 20 percent of how long we'll live. In other words, no matter how well you take care of yourself, you may be at greater risk for illnesses such as cardiovascular disease or diabetes than people from different genetic backgrounds (see Secret 11, page 79).

Also, the diet of many Blue-Zoners revolves around fresh, easily accessible, local foods not always obtainable elsewhere. The *marañón* fruit enjoyed in Nicoya, for example, contains five times more vitamin C than an orange, but is too fragile to be shipped in large quantities.

All of the Blue Zones, except the one in Loma Linda, California (which owes its existence to a religious tradition), place an emphasis on locally farmed foods. This close-to-the-land lifestyle is rapidly dying out, and it is possible that a switch to mass-produced food will impact the longevity of the people in these areas.

Finally, it is easy to talk about avoiding stress, but it remains a culturally conditioned affliction. The Blue Zones tend to promote levels of stress avoidance that are less common in the rest of the world and often difficult to re-create out of context.

Share in the Secret

Unfortunately, you can't just buy a one-way ticket to the Nicoya Peninsula and expect to live into your hundreds. Regardless of where you are, however, you can use the lessons learned from Ricardo's daily routine in your own life: Enjoy a healthy diet high in nutrients and low in calories; don't overeat; maintain a supportive social network; stay busy; exercise regularly; and avoid stress.

For example, eat more beans (from the Costa Rican diet) or tofu (from the Okinawan diet). You can also try eating larger lunches and smaller dinners as a way of restricting calories. Although your family may not be as cohesive as the ones in Loma Linda or Sardinia, you can widen your social circle by volunteering or taking up a sport or hobby. Aside from providing large support networks, these activities will also help you form a *plan de vida* to keep you active, motivated, and stress-free.

It's virtually impossible to create a Blue Zone in your hometown, because they are so largely dependent on genetic, cultural, environmental, and other factors as yet unknown. But there is no reason that new ones cannot come into being. As Buettner says, "Encoded in the world's Blue Zones are centuries—even millennia—of human experiences. I believe that it's no coincidence that the way these people eat, interact with each other, shed stress, heal themselves, avoid disease, and view their world yields them more good years of life.... To learn from them, we need only be open and ready to listen."

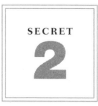

Brewer's Yeast

BARBARA PRITZKAT

ecause a mouse drank Coca-Cola and lost its fur, Barbara
Pritzkat eats yeast.

Back in the 1940s and '50s, Barbara discovered the work
of Adelle Davis, a pioneer in nutrition and health, then a
relatively new field. Promoting a diet of unprocessed whole foods
combined with intelligent dietary supplementation, Davis's bestselling
books, including *Let's Eat Right to Keep Fit,* influenced both the public
and a great number of researchers.

Barbara, who in 1947 had just graduated from UCLA with a degree
in engineering, was a neighbor of Davis's in Palos Verdes, California,
and was introduced to her work when Davis gave a series of lectures at
a local high school. Barbara was immediately hooked on her ideas about
nutrition, particularly after watching a demonstration in which Davis fed
cola to one mouse and water to another. Over the course of a few weeks,

the cola-drinking mouse lost its fur and began to look sickly. At the time, most people thought Coca-Cola was harmless, or even good for you. (Davis helped the sickly mouse regain its health and fur; no animals were harmed in the conducting of her experiment.)

Barbara was already predisposed to eating well because her father, a promising editor at MGM film studios in the 1920s, had died at thirty-five of a stroke brought on by alcoholism and the enormous pressure of the movie business. Barbara and her husband, Marty, chose Davis's healthier lifestyle, keeping clear of preservatives, refined sugars, and processed foods, and instead eating whole foods whenever possible. "The kids didn't even know about soft drinks until they saw them at other people's houses."

At the core of Davis's program is brewer's yeast, an excellent source of B vitamins, which Barbara and Marty take in powder form dissolved in water each morning. They never miss a morning, even when they travel—which in Barbara's case is frequently. Back in the 1970s, spurred in part by the international interest in King Tut's tomb, Barbara started taking a correspondence course in ancient art at UCLA. At first she studied for fun, but she slowly became serious about the subject; in 1982, at age fifty-six, she received a certificate in archeology. She then began working at excavations, first in Costa Rica and then, for the past dozen years, at a dig called Tel Mozan at the ancient Palace of Urkesh, located in a flat, arid valley north of the Great Syrian Desert on the border of Iraq and Syria. She works primarily as a surveyor, using her engineering skills in helping the diggers locate their targets.

Lately she is thinking of retiring because she imagines her team finds it embarrassing to have an eighty-three-year-old surveyor among them. The team members don't agree at all, pointing out that her stamina and health are as good as or better than anyone else's on the dig—despite the fact that she spends many weeks each year rising at 5 A.M. to work among scorpions in 110-degree temperatures, all while completely draped in long garments in deference to local Muslim culture and drinking impure water.

The Facts on Brewer's Yeast

A group of single-celled fungi that break sugars down into alcohol and release carbon dioxide, yeasts have been known to humankind for eons. Although not all types are useful and some can cause infections in people, the species *Saccharomyces cerevisiae,* or brewer's yeast, has helped people make bread and beverages since before the advent of recorded history.

The earliest records of beer making, dating back six thousand years to ancient Sumer, indicate that people possessed rudimentary knowledge about how to maintain colonies of S. *cerevisiae* to pass from one batch of beer to the next. Alcohol making became more sophisticated as it moved to Egypt and eventually to Europe, but people's understanding of fermentation remained limited: No one comprehended that yeast was made of living organisms. Theories abounded for what it was exactly that turned fruit and grains into alcohol. For example, an Old Norwegian term for yeast, *kveik,* is derived from the word for "kindling," reflecting the idea that yeast started a chemical "fire" that produces alcohol.

In seventeenth-century Paris, baking a baguette was considered sacrilegious. The devil was in the leavening. Because the functioning of yeast was still poorly understood, the only reliable source of it for baking was the foam skimmed from vats of fermenting beer. Problems arose when, based on a quote from Saint Paul in First Corinthians, the Paris Faculty of Medicine declared beer a "corrupt substance" and forbade it. Fortunately for the bakers, the public ignored the ban.

IF YOU CAN'T EAT IT . . .

As an added bonus to all of yeast's internal benefits, it's also a handy skin cream. Studies conducted at the University of Munich found that creams containing brewer's yeast were highly effective in treating acne, with 80 percent of participants reporting significant improvement over a five-month period.

It wasn't until the nineteenth century, when Louis Pasteur studied the properties of alcohol, that these misconceptions were laid to rest. In 1857, Pasteur published a paper titled "Notes on So-called Lactic Fermentation," in which he identified yeast as a new type of organism and established fermentation as the biological process through which it converted sugar to alcohol.

Although yeast is more valued for its ability to ferment food and drink than for its nutrients, people have long been marginally aware of its health benefits. Even in the Middle Ages, infants were often fed the yeasty sediment from cloudy beers as a way to keep them healthy. These popular uses were given scientific grounding in the 1950s, when nutritionist Davis held forth on brewer's yeast, writing: "Yeast contains almost no fat, starch, or sugar; its excellent protein sticks to your ribs, satisfies the appetite, increases your basal metabolism, and gives you pep to work off unwanted pounds."

Yeast cells usually replicate through a process of asexual reproduction called budding, in which a parent cell divides and produces a daughter cell. In this way, each cell creates millions of offspring during its life cycle, requiring a great deal of energy and vitamins that aren't contained in the simple sugars they feed on. To solve this problem, the yeast cells manufacture their own B vitamins, proteins, and trace minerals. All of these nutrients are beneficial to human health.

The most important of these nutrients are the water-soluble B vitamins, including thiamine, riboflavin, niacin, vitamin B_6, pantothenic acid, folic acid, and biotin. Just one tablespoon of a good brand of brewer's yeast meets the recommended daily allowance for most of them. Without these vitamins, the body would not be able to metabolize the carbohydrates, fats, and proteins essential for growth; they are also essential for the maintenance of healthy hair, skin, nerves, blood cells, hormone-producing glands, and the immune system; a deficiency in any one of them can result in diseases like beriberi, pellagra, and anemia.

Another benefit of B vitamins is that they keep homocysteine levels low. Homocysteine is an amino acid present in human blood that is

DOCTOR LIQUOR

◆

Alcohol is one of humanity's oldest tonics, dating back to the ancient Sumerians, who described the feeling it induces as "exhilarated, wonderful, and blissful," and the Egyptians, who were among the first to turn grapes into wine. They passed this tradition on to the Greeks, who in turn introduced it across the Mediterranean. By approximately 500 B.C., the Romans had adopted both viticulture and drinking wine as cultural institutions.

Over the ensuing centuries, scientists began to take an interest in alcohol's life-extending properties: They noticed that when animal remains or plant matter were left in distilled spirits, they didn't rot. If simple life forms could be preserved in this *quinta essentia* (Latin for "quintessence," or "fifth element," to go with air, earth, fire, and water), they reasoned, mightn't it preserve human life? "We call it aqua vitae, and this name is remarkably suitable, for it is really a water of immortality," wrote Arnaud de Villeneuve, a thirteenth-century French professor. "It prolongs life, clears away ill humors, revives the heart, and maintains youth."

Alcohol's potential medicinal uses were eclipsed by its inebriating qualities, however, which in the United States led to the passage of the Volstead Act of 1919, banning the sale and consumption of alcohol.

Prohibition was repealed in 1933, and American views on alcohol have continued to liberalize. This trend has been aided by medical discoveries suggesting that the ancients were on to something: When consumed in moderation, alcohol does offer health benefits. An extensive research review by the National Institute on Alcohol Abuse and Alcoholism determined that moderate drinking increases longevity and decreases the risk of heart disease by 25 to 50 percent in men

strongly influenced by people's diets. Epidemiological studies have linked high levels of homocysteine to stroke, coronary heart disease, and peripheral vascular disease.

Yeast also provides protein—a single (two-ounce) serving of debittered brewer's yeast, 40 to 50 percent protein by weight, offers 8 grams of protein and 1 gram of fat for just 58 calories.

and 20 to 40 percent in women. Other studies have shown that moderate drinkers undergo fewer hospitalizations and have fewer disabilities than do the general population, and that moderate drinkers who do suffer certain kinds of heart attack are 32 percent less likely to die of their illness than nondrinkers—as well as 59 percent less likely to have another attack.

One of the healthiest types of alcohol is red wine. Aside from the cardiovascular benefits inherent in its alcohol content, it also contains polyphenolic flavonoids, such as resveratrol, quercetin, and catechins. These substances, found in grape skins, act as antioxidants. Not only are flavonoids believed to fight off illnesses such as cancer and Alzheimer's disease, but recent research also suggests that resveratrol specifically may fight obesity and slow aging.

Despite all the positive research, experts remain uncertain whether or not moderate drinking is a cause of better health or simply a habit of healthy people. And it's easy to get too much of a good thing. The *Dietary Guidelines for Americans* defines moderate drinking as one drink per day for women and two drinks per day for men. ("One drink" equals 12 fluid ounces of regular beer, 5 fluid ounces of wine, or 1.5 fluid ounces of 80 proof distilled spirits.) Beyond this limit, alcohol consumption ceases to be regenerative and becomes a degenerative force. Alcohol abuse can lead to liver cirrhosis, anemia, peptic ulcers, bleeding disorders, and heart failure. (In addition, alcohol-related accidents account for roughly 40 percent of all traffic fatalities in the United States each year.)

Considering these risks, alcohol's modern-day advocates may be giving the brew more credit than it deserves. Still, although alcohol doesn't hold the key to eternal life, for most, moderate drinking is enjoyable and helps relieve stress, which is a health boost in and of itself (see Secret 22, page 166).

Finally, brewer's yeast is also a good source of trace minerals, including selenium, copper, iron, zinc, potassium, magnesium, and chromium, all important for good health.

Despite all its benefits, brewer's yeast is not a cure-all. Its long history as a health supplement has contributed to the perpetuation of myriad medical myths, such as its alleged ability to relieve anxiety, ease carpal tunnel syndrome, cure constipation, combat anemia, improve physical performance, and keep fleas off your dog. Don't expect it to work on these issues.

Furthermore, brewer's yeast isn't always the best way to obtain many of the vitamins and minerals that it offers. For example, the unprocessed yeast doesn't contain vitamin B_{12}; this nutrient must be added, so the amount will vary depending on the type of brewer's yeast you use, as well as how long it has been sitting on the shelf. In fact, the vitamin content of all yeasts varies, because the methods used to cultivate each yeast (that is, the types of foods on which they are raised) affect its nutrient content.

Another downside is the taste—many people simply can't abide it. Others suffer adverse gastrointestinal reactions. As Davis herself writes, "Just as you may not have enjoyed your first taste of coffee, you may not enjoy your introduction to yeast... In case your digestion is below par, yeast may blow you up like a zeppelin."

To avoid a zeppelin belly, Davis and others recommend that newcomers start by taking a small amount until their systems become accustomed to it.

Share in the Secret

Three different types of *S. cerevisiae* fall under the category of brewer's yeast. The first is active yeast used to make beer or wine. Although it contains the same nutrients as other yeast cultures, this form is living and shouldn't be ingested as a supplement.

The second type is a by-product of beer brewing and winemaking that has been deactivated, or killed through heating; this is the type most often sold as a supplement under the name brewer's yeast. Bitter and nutty tasting, extracts of this yeast type are made into Vegemite and Marmite, the spreads beloved by many Australians.

The third type of supplemental yeast is termed nutritional yeast and has been developed for those who dislike the taste of brewer's yeast. It is the same species, but instead of being harvested from alcohol production it is grown on a molasses-based medium or on sugar beets, a process that mitigates the bitter taste imparted to yeasts cultivated in beer.

Although it can be taken in pill form, many prefer to use yeast as a condiment. *The Encyclopedia of Healing Foods* offers these suggestions to yeast up your diet:

- Sprinkle a tablespoon of brewer's yeast over hot or cold cereals.

- Mix it into soups or sauces. The taste goes especially well with split pea soup or any dish made with tomato sauce.

- Place a tablespoonful into baked goods.

- Sprinkle it on popcorn in place of salt.

- Sprinkle a spoonful over cottage cheese or yogurt.

PEP UP WITH PEP-UP

◆

For the more adventurous, Adelle Davis created a breakfast drink she dubbed Pep-Up. Here is a recipe from her multimillion-copy–selling 1954 classic, *Let's Eat Right to Keep Fit*

1 quart skim, low-fat, or whole milk, preferably medically certified raw

1 teaspoon to ½ cup yeast (depending on whether you are a beginner or a veteran yeast fan)

¼ to ½ cup powdered milk (not instant)

1 tablespoon soy, peanut, or safflower oil or mixed vegetable oils

½ teaspoon magnesium oxide

1 tablespoon granular lecithin (more if blood cholesterol is above 180 milligrams per 100 cc)

1 or 2 eggs, as desired

½ cup frozen, undiluted orange juice or ½ cup apricot nectar or grape juice or ½ banana or 3 or 4 tablespoons chunk pineapple or frozen berries or any strong-flavored fruit

Put everything together in a blender or food processor, mix well, and drink.

Caloric Reduction

GEORGE BURNS

The name Nathan Birnbaum may not mean much to you, but the alias he picked when he entered show business—George Burns—was a familiar one for the ten decades in which he performed. One of twelve children, Burns started singing when he was a child, quitting school in the fourth grade to make it a profession. He was doing a solo vaudeville act—singing, dancing, and telling jokes—when he met Grace Ethel Cecile Rosalie Allen, a young Irish Catholic singer; soon after, the two realized they worked better together than on their own and became Burns and Allen, one of the most famous comedy teams of the twentieth century.

The act became successful: They moved from second to top billing, landed a radio show, and then, in the 1950s, a high-rated, long-running eponymous television program. Burns's television production company was equally successful, churning out many hits, from *The Bob Cummings Show* to *Mr. Ed*.

After Gracie died in 1964 at age sixty-nine, Burns scaled back his roles until 1975, when he appeared in the movie *The Sunshine Boys* (a part that his best friend, Jack Benny, who had recently died, was to have played). Burns won an Oscar for his role and went on to guest-star in such movies as 1977's *Oh God!* (when asked how he landed the title role, he replied, "I was the closest to Him in age"), *Sergeant Pepper's Lonely Hearts Club Band* (1978), and *18 Again!* (1988), in which he played an eighty-one-year-old, although he had just celebrated his ninety-second birthday.

Burns died in 1996, just after his hundredth birthday. He was remarkably healthy, outliving nearly all his contemporaries. About his advanced age, he once remarked, "I get a standing ovation just standing."

Burns was also the author of ten bestselling books. His literary agents, Richard Pine and his father, Arthur Pine, used to travel to Los Angeles for a yearly lunch with Burns at the Hillcrest Country Club. Even when Burns was approaching ninety, he looked remarkably healthy. After lunch he would play cards, take a nap, go about his day, meet friends for dinner.

"Whenever I saw him," Richard remembers, "I was always a little in awe and a little in heaven. My father was more at ease. Once, during one of these lunches, he was looking at Burns and how robust he was when he suddenly asked, out of the blue, 'George, how do you stay so fit and healthy? What's your advice?'

"There was the pause. Burns took a puff from his ever-present cigar, exhaled, and said in his gravelly voice, 'Eat half.'"

> "KEEPING OFF *a large weight loss is a phenomenon about as common in American medicine as an impoverished dermatologist.*"
>
> — CALVIN TRILLIN, AMERICAN JOURNALIST, HUMORIST, AND FOOD WRITER

The Facts on Caloric Reduction

While much of the world doesn't have enough to eat, people living in developed countries can have too much. Obesity is an epidemic in many Western nations, including the United States, where in 2009 it was estimated that 33 percent of the population was overweight and even more—34 percent—was obese.

So while countless people are looking for food, many people in the West are looking to stop eating so much of it. Some do it for vanity—few people in our culture prefer being fat. Some do it for health reasons, because being overweight can cause a litany of illnesses, from cancer to stroke. And some do it for longevity, as a burst of new research supports calorie reduction as a lifespan extender.

"I KEEP MY HEALTH by dieting. People gorge themselves with rich foods, use up their time, ruin their digestion, and poison themselves. . . . If the doctors would prescribe dieting instead of drugs, the ailments of normal man would disappear. Half the people are food drunk all the time. That is the secret of my health."

~THOMAS EDISON, AMERICAN INVENTOR

Perhaps the first person to write about eating less for better health was Luigi Cornaro, who, as mentioned in the introduction, reduced his food intake to twelve to fourteen ounces a day of solid foods and fourteen ounces of wine. He later reduced those amounts, and lived to be 102.

In the early twentieth century, a Newburgh, New York, doctor named William Jones reported that a fasting spider will live longer than one that eats a normal diet. These findings were supported by studies at Cornell University in the 1930s showing that rats on a limited diet lived twice as long as other rats. Fifty years later, UCLA researchers released similar results involving mice; over the last decade, an increasing number of living creatures, from yeast to fish to dogs, have had their laboratory lives extended thanks to calorie restriction.

Additional research has indicated that eating less has positive effects on overall health: Recent studies at the University of Wisconsin have shown that calorie restriction can result in a reduced incidence of age-related disorders, including cardiovascular disease and diabetes, in monkeys, while another study at New York's Mount Sinai School of Medicine also found that monkeys on restricted diets were less likely to develop Alzheimer's disease.

The National Institute on Aging has conducted three pilot studies of calorie restrictions on humans called CALERIE, or the Comprehensive Assessment of Long-Term Effects of Reducing Intake of Energy, on 132 men and women around the country.

So far, the results of long-term testing of humans are inconclusive but promising. Several studies have indicated that a calorie-restricted diet in which participants eat up to 25 percent less than they would normally eat reduces overall cholesterol, LDL (bad) cholesterol, triglyceride levels, and blood pressure.

According to research from the Mayo Clinic, the following health benefits have been demonstrated for animals on a calorie-restricted diet:

- Rodents whose calorie consumption was reduced by 30 to 60 percent before the age of six months increased their maximum life span by 30 to 60 percent.

- Rodents subjected to a calorie reduction of 44 percent as adults increased their maximum life span by 10 to 20 percent.

- Rodents on a calorie-restricted diet developed fewer chronic diseases associated with aging or had delayed development of these diseases.

- A calorie-restricted diet decreased the deterioration of nerves in the brain and increased the creation of nerves in animals with neurobiological diseases, such as Alzheimer's, as well as in those that had suffered a stroke.

Despite these results, some researchers believe that a calorie-restricted diet merely triggers a survival mechanism in animals with already

FAD DIETS

◆

Not all diets are as strict as the calorie reduction diet. And some of them probably even work, especially those that require serious commitment and involve exercise as well. Scientifically unfounded fad diets, on the other hand, generally promise great results without much effort.

Nonetheless, fad diets have probably been around for as long as people have been overweight. No one knows exactly when they started, but we do know that William the Conqueror, king of England at the end of the eleventh century, was so obese that King Philip of France compared him to a pregnant woman. Offended, William apparently locked himself in a room, consuming nothing but alcohol in hope of losing his belly.

It didn't work; when William died in 1087, the clergy were barely able to fit his bulky corpse into his stone sarcophagus. (Oddly, a drinking-man's diet returned to vogue in the 1960s—and was about as effective then as it had been nine hundred years earlier.)

Over the centuries, weight-loss schemes became more sophisticated but no more useful. In 1820, for example, a vinegar-and-water diet swept Europe, but after many years of popularity, it died off, as did the later theories of Horace Fletcher, aka the Great Masticator. Fletcher proclaimed that it didn't matter *what* you ate as long as you chewed each mouthful thirty-two times. Aside from promoting weight loss, this method was supposed to make

short life spans, such as rodents, thus allowing them to outlive food shortages; these experts say it's unclear whether people, who already live eight decades or more, will see similar benefits from a calorie-restricted diet.

And there's a darker side to eating less: You must guard against undernourishment. In general, calorie-restricted diets involve eating 20 to 30 percent fewer calories while taking in the same amount of nutrients as before. This means that you must be careful about your food choices, as several studies have shown that unsupervised calorie restriction can lead to many ills, including muscle loss, hormonal changes, fatigue, its practitioners stronger and less prone to constipation.

In the early twentieth century, vendors of patent medicines sold pills purported to contain tapeworms, which, once established in the gut, were said to help their hosts fight the urge to overeat. Despite the fact that the pills probably never contained tapeworms at all (not that you would really want one), stories of people ingesting the ravenous creatures still crop up today: Perhaps the world's most famous tapeworm was the one rumored to have lived inside opera singer Maria Callas.

Smoking was another unlikely twentieth-century fad diet. Tobacco company Brown and Williamson claimed that its Kool cigarettes kept people's waists slim, their heads clear, and their bodies protected against colds. Similarly, in 1925, the manufacturer of Lucky Strikes urged dieting smokers to "Reach for a Lucky instead of a sweet."

Cigarette companies weren't the only ones trying to create a mass demand for their products. In 1934, the United Fruit Company endorsed the work of Dr. George Harrop, who promoted a diet consisting of skim milk and bananas. Other modern fad diets also have been composed primarily of a single food, such as cabbage soup, grapefruit, lemons, or chicken soup.

Perhaps the most difficult diet to follow is also the one that offers the fastest results (at least in terms of weight loss): the air diet. "Breatharians" believe that food and even water may not be necessary; instead, they maintain that humans can survive by ingesting only *prana*, the vital life force of the universe.

diarrhea, reduced bone density, gallstones, and, not surprisingly, irritability. Imagine how a dog feels when most of his meal is taken away. Humans can react similarly.

Furthermore, not all researchers on calorie restriction have come to the same conclusion: Some of their work has failed to show any benefit, and other scientists have wondered if the positive results derived not from the subjects consuming fewer calories, but from some other aspect of minimal eating. For example, high-calorie diets can cause an imbalance in gut bacteria, while low-calorie diets do not; however, many believe there might be better ways to avoid that proliferation.

There is also the issue of whether caloric restriction must begin at a young age to be effective or can begin at any time and still produce results.

And finally, the fact remains that very few people are willing to eat only half the food on their plates. They want it all.

Share in the Secret

If George Burns could do it, so can you. But be careful. If you decide to restrict calories, make sure that what you do eat is nutritionally dense. Simply eating limited-calorie meals of diet sodas and celery isn't going to give you the vitamins and minerals you'll need during your day.

And consider vitamins and supplements if your carefully planned diet doesn't include everything you need to stay healthy.

"A FULL BELLY *is the mother of all evil.*"

~BENJAMIN FRANKLIN, AMERICAN STATESMAN AND INVENTOR

According to Susan Roberts, professor at the Friedman School of Nutrition Science and Policy at Tufts University and author of *The "I" Diet,* her study of caloric reduction calls for a 25 percent cut in calories, but she believes it can be done in any way the dieter wishes as long as it feels comfortable—eating a full diet one day and then cutting calories the next, or eating a normal meal once a day with a reduced meal at other times. Still, she says she would personally put her bet on consistent everyday calorie reduction as the best route.

Here are some tips from the Calorie Restriction Society, founded in 1993:

- *Avoid simple sugars and flours.* Sugars and flours generally contain very little nutrition for their calorie content. They also have high glycemic indices, which means that your body absorbs them quickly, leaving you wanting more a short time later.

- *Eat both green leafy (salad) and other, nonleaf vegetables.* Vegetables contain the highest content of a wide variety of nutrients for

24

GEORGE BURNS'S EAT-LESS MENU

◆

Burns wrote down his supposed diet in his book *How to Live to Be 100—Or More* in 1983. What's really funny is how many people today might pick it up and think he was serious.

BREAKFAST

1 small glass orange juice

Bowl bran cereal with milk

2 cups coffee, black

I let the cereal soak in the milk so it gets a little soggy. That way it doesn't make a noise when I'm eating, because I'm too tired from taking bows the night before.

LUNCH

Bowl of canned salmon with white vinegar and lemon

1 English muffin, toasted

1 cup coffee, black

English muffins usually come sliced in half horizontally. I like each half sliced the same way, so the muffin is in four slices. That way I eat two slices and wind up eating just half a muffin.

DINNER

Bowl of soup

Mixed green salad

Broiled fish

Two vegetables

1 slice bread, buttered

1 cup coffee, black

Ice cream

If it's white fish, then I have green vegetables. Green and white go together beautifully. But if the fish is red snapper, then I don't have green vegetables. I have yellow squash, even though I hate yellow squash. I can't stand a meal where the colors clash.

their calorie content of any food group. By volume (and often by calories), vegetables are the major component of many calorie-restricted but not nutrient-deficient diets.

• *Carefully select your protein and fat sources.* Both protein and fat are required macronutrients, but their form can have a significant influence on a person's risk factors for a wide variety of diseases.

• *Make sure your protein intake is sufficient but not overly abundant.* Common recommendations for total protein intake range from 0.6 to 0.8 grams per kilogram of body weight, and some recommendations are much higher. This is probably a minimum.

• *Select monounsaturated fats, avoid saturated fats, and consume some omega-3 fats.* Foods containing monounsaturated fats include olive oil, almonds, hazelnuts, and avocados. Most of your fat intake should be from these foods. A very small amount of fat should be in the form of omega-3 fatty acids, which are found in fatty fish (salmon, for example) and flax oil. Caution: Fatty foods, even healthy choices, are high in calories, so be sure that you carefully track your intake so as to stay within your calorie goal.

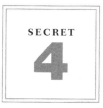
Chicken Soup

MY SIXTH-GRADE TEACHER

When I was in elementary school, the highlight of any year was the arrival of a substitute teacher. Unfamiliar with the students, helpless to control the class much less assign any work, the frazzled and unhappy sub represented the closest thing we had to a day off while still sitting in a classroom.

Unfortunately, no student of Mrs. Goddell got that privilege. A tough, old-fashioned teacher, she kept us students waiting for the day she didn't show up. As far as I know, Mrs. Goddell never missed a day of school in her life. She once said that she'd never missed one as a student, either, meaning she'd spent six decades never being sick, despite spending every workday exposed to countless kids' coughs and sneezes. Outside of health care workers, few people spend more time among the ill than teachers.

The first time I stayed home sick while enrolled in her sixth-grade class, I came in the next day still coughing and blowing my nose. She instructed me to eat chicken soup. When I asked why, she explained that consuming several bowls of chicken soup a week prevents colds. She'd learned this from her mother, who'd learned it from *her* mother, who for all I know heard it from many generations of chicken-soup eaters.

Once, at lunch hour, I caught her eating soup at her school desk from a china bowl she must have brought from home. The steamy soup's aroma, brimming with spices, chicken, and vegetables, lingered all afternoon, leading us to hope that the soup's appearance meant she was about to take ill. Dream on, she would have told us.

The Facts on Chicken Soup

Chicken soup has probably been part of the human diet for as long as there have been chickens and soup. It was prescribed for colds in ancient Egypt, and continued to be considered a powerful remedy from antiquity through the Middle Ages. Tenth-century Persian physician Avicenna was an advocate, as was the twelfth-century Jewish physician Moses Maimonides, who also recommended it for people suffering from hemorrhoids, constipation, and leprosy. Chicken soup eventually became known as "Jewish penicillin."

Through the years, doctors and mothers alike have recommended chicken soup, despite the lack—until recently—of scientific proof of its efficacy. As reported in 2000 in the medical magazine *Chest,* researchers at the University of Nebraska Medical Center found that the mixture of vitamins and nutrients in chicken soup has an anti-inflammatory effect, slowing the growth of the white blood cells called neutrophils, which stimulate the release of mucus. Fewer neutrophils equals fewer cold symptoms.

Similarly, according to UCLA School of Medicine pulmonary specialist Irwin Ziment, MD, chicken soup contains druglike agents that resemble those found in modern cold medicines. For example, an amino

THE CHICKEN OR THE SOUP?

◆

Another line of research into chicken soup indicates that the chicken may not matter as much as the rest of the soup. Some spices, such as curry, pepper, and garlic, can help ease a cough by thinning mucus; these flavorings have been used for centuries to treat respiratory diseases due to their various antibiotic, antiviral, and antifungal properties.

And when chicken soup contains vegetables such as onions, carrots, turnips, celery, and parsley, the brew is a potential panacea. Onions, for example, contain protein, calcium, sulfur (which itself contains compounds with anti-inflammatory properties and the antibiotic oil allicin), and several vitamins including C, E, the B complex, and A, the last of which helps fight off infections by enhancing the actions of white blood cells that destroy harmful bacteria and viruses. Carrots are an excellent source of beta-carotene, which the body converts to vitamin A. Turnips, too, are rich in beta-carotene and protect mucous membranes (especially in the lungs and intestinal tract) from cancer cells and free-radical damage. Celery has long been used to promote restfulness and sleep, important factors in fighting a cold, and its high iron and magnesium content are beneficial to blood cells. Moreover, due to its antispasmodic properties, celery is beneficial for lung conditions, including asthma and bronchitis. And finally, parsley contains two components that seem to provide health benefits: volatile oils and flavonoids, a type of polyphenol.

acid released from chicken during cooking chemically resembles the drug acetylcysteine, prescribed for bronchitis and other respiratory ailments.

New Japanese research, published in the *Journal of Agricultural and Food Chemistry*, shows that chicken soup may even fight high blood pressure, because chicken breasts contain collagen proteins, which display effects similar to ACE inhibitors, the most popular medications for treating high blood pressure. Researcher Ai Saiga and his colleagues tested the chicken-based collagen on laboratory rats and reported finding significant and prolonged decrease in blood pressure.

Finally, the steam from chicken soup opens up congested noses and chests, which is why for centuries doctors have recommended hot liquids, from simple water to complicated stews, to alleviate cold symptoms.

The bottom line: There is no absolute proof that chicken soup can prevent a cold, but there is plenty of evidence that it can alleviate its symptoms. Its other powers are still being investigated.

Share in the Secret

If you want to feel healthy right now, cook up a big vat of soup.

CHICKEN SOUP

This recipe, from *Cooking Jewish,* by Judy Bart Kancigor, was created by Judy's mother. "It is dark golden in color," Kancigor writes, "intensely flavorful, and, in short, an elixir of the gods."

2 chickens (3½ to 4 pounds each) with necks and gizzards but no liver, quartered

2 pounds carrots (yes, 2 pounds, not 2 carrots)

2 large onions, cut in half

5 large ribs celery with leaves, cut in half

2 large parsnips

1 small sweet potato (6 ounces), cut in half

1 turnip (6 ounces), cut in half

1 rutabaga (6 ounces), cut in half

1 small celery root, cut in half (optional)

½ large green bell pepper, stemmed and seeded

½ large yellow pepper, stemmed and seeded

2 large bunches dill, coarsely chopped (about 1½ cups)

½ bunch curly-leaf parsley, coarsely chopped (about ¼ cup)

3 cloves garlic

Kosher (coarse) salt and freshly ground black pepper to taste

Chopped dill, for serving (optional)

1. Place the chickens in a 16-quart stockpot and add water to barely cover. Bring just to the boiling point, then reduce the heat to a simmer and skim off the foam that rises to the top. Add all the remaining ingredients (except the optional chopped dill) and only enough water to come to within about two-thirds of the height of the vegetables in the pot. (Most recipes will tell you to add water to cover. Do not do this! You want elixir of the gods or weak tea? As the soup cooks, the vegetables will shrink and will be covered soon enough. Eight to 10 cups of water, total, is plenty for this highly flavorful brew.) Simmer, covered, until the chicken is cooked through, about 1½ hours.

2. Remove the chicken and about half the carrots; set aside.

3. Strain the soup through a fine-mesh strainer into another pot or container, pressing on the vegetables to extract all the flavor. Scrape the underside of the strainer with a rubber spatula and add the pulp to the soup. Discard the fibrous vegetable membranes that remain in the strainer. If you're fussy about clarity, you can strain the soup again through a fine tea strainer, but there goes some of the flavor. Cover the soup and refrigerate overnight.

4. When you are ready to serve the soup, scoop the congealed fat off the surface and discard it. Reheat, adding more dill if desired (and I do). Slice the reserved carrots, add them to the soup, and serve.

YIELD: *Makes about 3 quarts.*

CAN YOU HAVE TWO COLDS AT ONCE?

Research says yes. Most common colds are caused by something called a rhinovirus, of which there are many strains. Not only can you catch more than one of them simultaneously, if the two viruses invade the same cell at the same time, their DNA can apparently combine and produce an entirely new type of cold virus, using your cells as its incubator.

However, as science has only recently confirmed that this kind of activity is going on, there are no data yet on whether this new cold combination will give you worse symptoms than the cold or two you already have.

The good news: You can kill three colds with one stone. Once you've caught these viruses, your body will cure you by manufacturing virus-specific antibodies that then remain in your immune system, ready to fight off the new type of cold along with its two parents should they ever try to attack again.

HOLD THE SALT

◆

The most common seasoning people put in their chicken soup is salt. But doing so may negate the soup's benefits.

A little background: Salt, or sodium chloride, is the only type of rock that humans eat regularly—and have been doing so for millennia. Archeologists have found evidence that it's been harvested for at least eight thousand years; we know that nearly all ancient cultures eventually found ways to mine and/or trade for it.

Salt remained a highly prized commodity until the seventeenth century, when better mining drills and the development of geology revealed that salt could be found throughout nature. Since then, the problems associated with it involve overabundance rather than scarcity.

Salt is vital for human functioning: It helps maintain the fluid balance within cells, regulates blood pressure, transports nutrients and oxygen, and transmits nerve impulses in the form of electrical currents. Without it, the body would be unable to digest food, rid its cells of waste, regulate blood pressure, or engage and relax its muscles.

Because salt is ubiquitous—found in almost all foods—it's easy to fulfill our daily sodium requirement by eating a balanced diet. The problem is that most people eat far too much of it. The most common effect of this overconsumption is high blood pressure (hypertension). Hypertension makes the heart work harder, increasing the risk of heart disease and stroke; according to the World Health Organization, in 2003 hypertension caused about 4.5 percent of the current global disease burden.

A 2009 Centers for Disease Control (CDC) study concluded that the average person should consume no more than 1,500 milligrams of sodium per day. However, typical intake is currently estimated to be more than double that. A study reported in the New England Journal of Medicine in February, 2010 concluded that salt reduction by three grams per day in the average diet could prevent forty-four thousand deaths per year.

Still, one gram of salt is not as easy to cut out as it sounds. Only 11 percent of the sodium that Americans ingest comes from salt in the shaker or is added during cooking. Most of the rest is packed into processed foods. Some approximate amounts:

- Canned chicken noodle soup (one cup): 1,100 milligrams

- Cottage cheese (one cup, 1 percent milk fat): 900 milligrams

- Canned vegetarian vegetable soup (one cup): 800 milligrams

- Canned sweet corn (one cup): 575 milligrams

- Bagel (one medium, plain, onion, poppy, or sesame): 400 milligrams

Nevertheless, salt can't be blamed for all high-blood-pressure problems. According to the American Heart Association, the direct causes of up to 90 percent of high blood pressure cases are unknown. Many other factors—including obesity, lack of exercise, genetic predisposition, excessive alcohol consumption, diabetes, kidney disease, and old age—play a contributing role. New research also indicates that a large percentage of adults seem able to consume excess salt without its affecting their blood pressure. And, as nearly all the research concerning salt's effects on health is heart related, it's not yet clear how an overabundance of salt affects the rest of the body.

However, based on what science now knows, excess salt is probably dangerous, so when you're seasoning that chicken soup, think about pepper, basil, thyme, bay leaves, garlic, parsley, rosemary—so many seasonings, so little salt.

Cold Showers

NATE HALSEY

N ate Halsey responds to a challenge. Over the course of his thirty-eight years, he has bungee jumped in South Africa, hang glided in the French Alps, and skydived in Colorado. (Bungee jumping scared him the most.) He has also rock climbed; scuba dived; run a twelve-person, two-hundred-mile relay race; taken part in five marathons; and completed a three-week Outward Bound canoeing course, including a three-day solo in which he didn't eat. He has biked the coast of Sweden, hiked to the base camp on Mount Everest, and visited fifty countries. (Today he travels mostly as a Boston-based business consultant, attempting to bring renewable energy to rural communities in developing countries.)

The one challenge that Nate found most difficult to conquer is the secret to his excellent health: Every day, before going to work, he takes a frigid shower.

He got the idea a decade ago from a German friend who had attended an old-fashioned boarding school, where every morning he and his classmates were forced to take cold showers as a form of discipline. The friend swore it was the reason he was never sick.

Nate, who sometimes did get sick, gave it a try. It was unpleasant: "The first shower was very painful. I got really tense, closed my eyes, and went in. The next day I didn't do it. It seemed like too much, but then I decided to challenge myself again, and again, and now it's a routine."

The point isn't to pamper. "It isn't an enjoyable experience. The enjoyment comes after the shower is over. No need to drink coffee— I'm totally invigorated. And it's ecologically sound—it doesn't require electricity or a hot water heater."

Nate believes that if you take a hot shower in the winter and then go outside in the cold, you are weakening your body because it has to burn that much more energy to regulate itself, thus weakening the immune system.

He also says it's excellent for his skin, which doesn't dry out as it did when he took hot showers. "An old friend told me that Paul Newman dipped his face in a bucket of ice-cold water several times every morning to keep his skin taut and healthy. I wouldn't mind looking like Paul Newman."

The Facts on Cold Showers

Think about it: Cold showers have been around a lot longer than hot ones. But they weren't always considered salubrious. They were the sole option.

The concept of hydrotherapy, or using water to treat disease, was common during the ancient Egyptian, Greek, and Roman civilizations; the ancient Greek physician Hippocrates prescribed natural spring waters for sickness. In the East for the last five thousand years, yoga practitioners have recommended cold water showers to boost immunity against colds; traditional Chinese medicine uses cold water for healing;

CLEANING THE HEAD

◆

It doesn't matter whether you take a cold or hot shower if you don't take care of your showerhead. According to a 2009 study published in the *Proceedings of the National Academies of Science,* millions of mycobacteria can be found within a shower fixture, solidly stuck in their own slime. The study discovered about 20 percent of all showerhead samples contained mycobacteria, at least a hundred times more than expected—a worrisome finding because strains of this bacteria can cause lung disease, and showerheads aerate bacteria, making them easy to inhale.

According to the researchers, this is probably not a concern for the average person, but people with weak immune systems might want to change their showerheads every six months.

and to this day, people of the Shinto faith in Japan stand under cold waterfalls as part of a meditative practice called *misogi.*

In the Western world, the person most famous for promoting cold water therapy was a German priest, Sebastian Kneipp, who, in the 1860s, claimed to have cured his terminal lung disease by taking baths in the icy Danube River. His eventual prescription centered on a regime of alternating hot and cold water baths; his book, *My Water Cure,* published in 1886, is still in print today. (In Norway, Kneipp is more famous for his bread recipe based on whole wheat: Kneipbrød.)

Others also promoted cold-water cures throughout the eighteenth and nineteenth centuries, from the Austrian farmer Vincent Priessnitz to the Englishman Sir John Floyer, who wrote *Psychrolousía; or, The History of Cold Bathing, Both Ancient and Modern.* One of the most famous recent champions of the cold shower is the fictional spy, James Bond, who always begins his shower with warm water but then turns it cold to finish. In the spa industry, this type of bathing is known as the Scottish shower.

Still, cold-water healing faded somewhat in the era of luxurious, well-appointed bathrooms. It is, however, making a comeback. Proponents claim that cold showers

- Improve circulation,

- Strengthen the skin,

- Bolster the immune system,

- Better your mood, and

- Invigorate the body.

Backing up these claims is a growing—but still rather small—body of scientific literature, much of it from northern Europe, home of cold-water therapy, where a 1987 study comparing a cold-shower group with a control group for six months found that the cold-shower group's colds were "significantly fewer, significantly milder, and slightly shorter."

Another study, performed in Prague, involved dunking physically fit young men in cold water to see if it would bolster immune response. The researchers found that doing so increased the white blood cell count, although they cautioned that the implications of their findings still needed to be studied. And at the medical school at Berlin's Humboldt University, doctors claim that exposing the body to regimens of intense heat followed by intense cold (as might be experienced by rolling in the snow after sitting in a sauna) increases resistance to chest infections.

Exposure to cold water may also increase levels of one of the body's natural antioxidants—glutathione—as a study of swimmers in Berlin found that exposure to ice-cold water elevated baseline levels of the substance. The researchers hypothesize that this is a form of "body hardening," a process in which the body adapts to certain stimuli (like cold water) by increasing its tolerance to stress. Whatever the case, year-round swimmers in Berlin (that is, the ones who take regular dips in freezing cold water during winter) suffer half as many chest infections as other people, say doctors at the Herzog-Julius Hospital in Bad Harzburg.

And although the cold shower has long been viewed as the ultimate libido killer, the truth may be exactly the opposite. A study by the Thrombosis Institute in London reported that, aside from health benefits like increased circulation, daily cold-water immersion stimulates the testicles to produce more sperm.

Still, cold showers have detractors. Says Dr. Rick Kellerman, chair of the Department of Family Medicine at the University of Kansas–Wichita School of Medicine: "The only reason I can think of to take a cold shower is the shock value to wake you up in the morning. I don't know of any American research that shows health benefits, but if I have a patient who takes one and says he feels better, I can't see any harm in it, except maybe a rare instance of getting too cold and short of breath, or if you have a heart condition."

Share in the Secret

Nate's best way to take a cold shower: Turn the water on for thirty seconds or so, dip your head in long enough to get it wet, turn off the water. Now that your hair is wet, wash it with shampoo. Lather it in. Turn on the water again. Return to the shower for less than thirty seconds, rinsing off your hair and wetting your skin. Turn the water off again, step out. Lather up with soap. Turn the water on again and jump in, rinsing off the soap. Turn the water off, step out. Put conditioner in your hair. Turn on the water, jump in, and rinse your body of the soap and conditioner.

The entire event should take about five minutes.

A few cautionary notes: Don't jump in all at once—this may hinder circulation. People who are extremely thin may not be able to tolerate cold showers; likewise, if you have any medical conditions, such as Reynaud's disease or blood pressure issues, talk to your doctor first. If you try a cold shower and don't warm up within a few minutes, consider a cold sponge bath instead.

Detoxification

PHILIP DAMON

Here's something few people can say: Phil Damon wakes every morning with sweet breath. He doesn't use deodorant. He doesn't change his socks or underwear every day. He has no body odor. Yet he showers only twice a week. (His wife verifies these claims.)

He credits detoxification.

Phil was born in 1937 in Chicago. His overweight father drank, smoked, and had a taste for rich food, dying at forty-five of complications of high blood pressure and a heart attack. His mother died at fifty of colon cancer. According to Phil, "they were examples of death by dietary misguidedness." But for the first part of his life, he followed in his parents' footsteps, except that he didn't smoke.

By the time Phil was thirty, he was overweight and suffering from terrible allergies; then, in 1969, he was diagnosed with melanoma and given a year to live. He survived the cancer, but went on to battle a miserable case of hemorrhoids. Reluctant to undergo a hemorrhoidectomy, he heeded the advice of a proctologist to cut out white flour and alcohol from his diet. Within two months, his symptoms disappeared. If it was possible to recover from hemorrhoids through diet alone, Phil wondered, what else was possible?

In the 1970s, Phil was teaching in Hawaii, which was teeming with seekers of holistic health and spiritual consciousness. He experimented with many different religious traditions and health practices, eventually finding a way to integrate a holistic way of life with spiritual self-awareness, as well as physical detoxification—the metabolic process by which the harmful qualities of a poison or toxin are reduced by the body. Detox, he says, allowed him to "return to something approaching a state of natural purity" in which the body can exercise its native intelligence and function as it has evolved to do: in harmony with nature.

Toxification—in which poisons accumulate in our bodies—is a passive as well as an active process. On one hand, we're all subjected to toxics (manmade poisons) and toxins (dangerous substances found in nature) over which we have little control: smokestack emissions, acid rain, pesticides, contaminated water. On the other hand, what we buy at the grocery store or eat at a restaurant is our choice, as are the products we use.

Phil's own detox regimen involved eating lean, fresh, and often raw foods: "The fattier, more processed, and more adulterated our diet, the greater amount of it is retained in our bodies. Organs are stressed by their efforts to eliminate the toxic molecules. The less concentrated the diet, the more efficiently this elimination takes place—from the blood through the bowels, bladder, lungs, and skin—so the toxics aren't retained in the cells."

When Phil, who now lives in Bellingham, Washington, first started, he says, "I cut out foods slowly. I still ate some meat, but no hot dogs, pork, fatty meats—only lean burgers on whole-wheat buns with lettuce and tomato and onion. I changed from white rice to brown rice (a big

COLONICS

◆

Colonic irrigation, also known as colon hydrotherapy, is the practice of flushing the colon with warm filtered water in order to loosen and remove accumulated waste. Colonic proponents believe that fecal matter sticks to the walls of the colon, hardens, impedes the organ's function, and leads to the absorption of toxins into the bloodstream through the colon walls. Think of it as the ultimate enema. (Enemas typically cleanse only the lower colon with one infusion of water; colonics clean the entire organ using multiple infusions.)

A typical session starts with the colon therapist inserting a speculum into the anus of the patient. The speculum is attached to a plastic hose leading to a hydrotherapy machine containing warm water (sometimes mixed with herbs or other liquids). After the water is pumped in, the colon responds by pushing the water and loosened feces out through the same tube in a reaction known as peristalsis.

The process usually lasts about an hour. Many people are willing to pay a great deal of money to have this done regularly. Does it do them any good? This is an open debate, but many doctors don't think so, and risks are involved, including the possibility that along with the bad you are flushing away the good—the friendly organisms that help your body thrive.

deal in Hawaii), and from white to whole-wheat flour." Soon sprouts became a major part of the diet as well—four ounces' worth, which he ate each evening before going to bed.

Putting the right things into his body was part of the battle. Over many years, Phil also tried detox fasts, most of them based on consuming only juice, as well as "dozens of week-long, twenty or more two-week, and about ten three-week ones, and several one-monthers" to detox his gut.

By taking enemas and the occasional colonic, he also claims to have detoxified his colon, even learning to do a shoulder stand with a quart of water in his colon "to facilitate the flush."

TOXIC CITY

◆

Toxins are everywhere: in the food we eat, the water we drink, the air we breathe. Luckily, they have little effect on us in small doses. However, when they accumulate in our bodies through repeated exposure, they can have serious effects. And their number is growing, due to the invention of new chemicals for industrial and scientific uses. The latest CDC *Report on Human Exposure to Environmental Chemicals* cataloged exposure levels to 212 separate toxins, 75 of which had never been measured before. This list includes a few toxins that are probably present in at least trace amounts in your body right now:

PHTHALATES

A class of compounds derived from phthalic acid with many common household uses

Sources: plastic softener, perfumes, hairsprays, lubricants, wood finishers, "new-car smell"

Dangers: cancer; phthalates also inhibit sexual development of male babies in utero

POLYCHLORINATED BIPHENYLS (PCBs)

A group of compounds used in the manufacture of many industrial items from plastics to insulation

Sources: fish, soil, drinking water, indoor air

Dangers: impairment of immune system and reproductive system, cancer, impairment of child neurological development

The Facts on Detoxification

Even as you read this book, all kinds of substances are coursing through your body that have no right to be there—and which, in sufficient quantity, could lead to disease. Ridding the body of these aliens is the principle behind detoxification.

These toxic substances include synthetic chemicals, metals, organic detritus, and/or unhealthy foods. And while there are almost as many different ways to detoxify as there are toxics and toxins, all call for a limitation on consumption or a purgation of things already consumed.

Detoxification is not a uniquely human concept. Most animals do it too. You'll often see a dog munching on some grass and vomiting shortly

FORMALDEHYDE

A colorless gas used primarily as a disinfectant and preservative

Sources: carpets, plastics, paper products, shampoos, bath products

Dangers: cancer

CARBAMATE INSECTICIDES, TRIAZINE HERBICIDES, AND NITRATES

Common pesticides

Sources: water supply

Dangers: detrimental effects on nervous, immune, and endocrine systems

DIOXINS

Toxic compounds usually occurring as waste products of industrial processes such as pesticide manufacture

Sources: dairy products, meat, fish, shellfish

Dangers: impairment of immune system, endocrine system, nervous system, and reproductive functions

HEAVY METALS

Metallic elements with specific gravity five or more times that of water, such as mercury, copper, arsenic, lead, cadmium, iron, and manganese

Sources: fish, contaminated water, soil, badly fitted fillings, lipstick (in the case of lead)

Dangers: headache, fatigue, anemia, dizziness, constipation, tremors, cancer

thereafter. This is doggie detox. Dogs' instincts (and intestines) tell them that the grass will make them throw up whatever surplus bile has been bothering them.

We aren't very different from dogs in this respect. Our impulse to vomit after ingesting poison, rancid food, or excessive alcohol is a crude but crucial detox method. In these situations, our internal detox system is overwhelmed, so we need to purge as much of the offending substance as we can, as quickly as possible.

Even before manmade toxins, such as chemical pesticides, came into existence, we still had to detoxify. For instance, you probably gag when tasting something particularly bitter or sour; this response—a kind of preventive detox—may be inherited from our hunter-gatherer days, when we had to worry much more about poisonous plants and animals that signaled us to keep away by emitting foul odors and tastes.

Keep in mind that your body is actually in a constant state of detoxification. Your liver, the largest internal organ, has many functions, including processing your blood, transforming toxins such as alcohol, drugs, and environmental pollutants into water-soluble substances that can be excreted

"A MAN TOO BUSY *to take care of his health is like a mechanic too busy to take care of his tools."* ~SPANISH PROVERB

(removed) in your urine or feces. The liver filters these bad guys out of the bloodstream at a rate of more than a quart of blood per minute. Your circulatory and lymphatic systems, meanwhile, transport toxic substances from every part of your body to your kidneys and liver, where they are either filtered and processed into waste or transformed and stored as a benign molecule in a fat cell.

Even without the threat of poison, we would still need to detoxify the toxins produced by our own bodies. These substances include hormones, chemicals that control body functions. Many things can stimulate hormone production, from the onset of menstruation to an invading bacterium to a sudden external threat. This last stimulus triggers the fight-or-flight response, during which a surge of hormones triggers a number of physiological changes geared toward physical alertness: Your heart races, your pupils dilate, and you start to think more intently and lucidly.

After the threat has passed, these hormones are swept out of your cells and removed from your bloodstream by your kidneys and liver. Otherwise, you'd remain in a state of permanent stress and quickly succumb to hypertension. This is just one example of how the body can produce something only temporarily beneficial. We need a method of clearing it, some way to reset; fortunately, our organs do that automatically.

If our bodies naturally and automatically detoxify, why have so many special programs claiming to optimize, maximize, or stimulate detoxification cropped up in the last few years? Has the world become more toxic?

44

Definitely. Many chemicals used commonly today were completely absent from our environment just a century ago. All have been linked to health problems—and all are commonly found in the bodies of adults in developed countries.

The toxins mentioned in the box (see page 42) aren't the only poisons in our systems. Science is constantly discovering more, which is why researchers in the new field of biomonitoring are attempting to study the human body's burden of environmental contaminants by measuring amounts in individuals' blood, urine, and tissues. For example, a study by the Mount Sinai School of Medicine in New York City found an average of ninety-one different chemicals in the bodies of research subjects; nearly all were known to be either toxic to the brain, carcinogenic, or teratogenic (causing birth defects). Though levels of these toxins tend to be infinitesimal, their cumulative and/or long-term effects concern scientists.

Hence the recent interest in various forms of detoxification. While plenty of research exists showing the dangers to humans and animals of a toxic environment, few long-term studies have been completed on the benefits of detoxification—in fact, no one really knows yet how well detox programs work, so be wary of any that offer you a guarantee. However, rates of diseases, including cancer and liver disease, that are linked to toxic exposures are increasing. If you decrease your body's level of synthetic chemicals, chances are good that your health will improve.

Share in the Secret

If you want to take extra steps to rid your body of toxins, your options are bountiful.

The most common way to detoxify is probably the least expensive: fasting. Countless fasting regimens exist; almost all of them require you to avoid meats, processed foods, and anything altered chemically or created with additives, as well as caffeine, alcohol, and nicotine. Make sure to read up on a fast before starting it. You need to make sure that what you're doing is healthy and appropriate. It's also a good idea to talk to your doctor.

One popular detox regimen prescribes an all-juice diet to help minimize toxins from the buildup of waste and fats in the colon. Unfortunately, if you are not consuming solid food, you will have to induce bowel movements by taking a laxative. Special teas, saltwater, and enemas are variously suggested as excellent ways to induce bowel movements and achieve colon irrigation.

Many liquid detox programs go even further in limiting consumption. The most famous of these is the Master Cleanse, which requires you to ingest nothing but lemon juice, maple syrup, cayenne pepper, and water for a period of time. This lemonadelike drink is supposed to supply all the nutrients that your body needs to operate, but many experts disagree, fearing that the lack of protein, vitamins, and minerals can be harmful.

Another common style of detox—often paired with some variation on fasting—focuses on purging the body through heat. Saunas and Bikram yoga (yoga practiced in a hot room) have long been touted as techniques for stimulating the release of toxics by inducing sweat and promoting blood flow. Now, researchers at the University of Toronto are studying far-infrared saunas, which apparently mimic the range of solar radiation. Naturopath Dr. Sat Dharam Kaur, who practices at the Trillium Healing Arts Center in Ontario, claims that one hundred hours of far-infrared sauna time can sweat out 80 percent of an adult's toxic body burden.

Similarly, cleansing mineral or homeopathic baths are often used to leach out toxins from the skin.

Be careful about the commercial products you select for your detox, however. Many people claim to have invented (usually expensive) detoxification systems that probably don't work. If those miracle cures advertised on late-night television were legitimate, you'd probably have heard of them by now. In England, the Medical Health Care Products Regulatory Agency has started investigating such claims, and a report by Voice of Young Science (VoYS), representing more than three hundred postgraduate and postdoctoral science students, found that no two companies use the same definition of *detox*, rendering their claims virtually meaningless.

FEED A COLD, STARVE A FEVER

For eons parents have given this advice to their children. Is it correct?

Possibly. A feverish flu requires that your body expend a great deal of energy in metabolic activity. So does digestion. The less you eat, the less you'll digest, and the better chance you'll give your body to marshal all its resources to fight off enemy germs.

Fighting a cold, however, doesn't use up the same resources, and because colds can be long lasting, you'll need all the antibodies you can create to fight them. These antibodies are built, in part, from the vitamin-rich foods you eat—in moderation.

Everything is open to interpretation, however. Some say the axiom is misunderstood, referring not to eating and drinking at all. Instead, the feed/starve metaphor refers to the body's temperature. "Starving" a fever means avoiding its most common causes—that is, to starve the body of anything that could cause a fever. "Feeding" a cold means trying to break into a sweat—that is, to feed it with warmth. Thus, the phrase "Feed a cold, starve a fever" suggests that to avoid all illnesses, we should bundle up and stay warm.

Another theory: In the past, having a cold wasn't dangerous, so victims were fed to help them survive the illness. But many feverish people were seriously ill and tended to die. So, the thinking went, why waste valuable food feeding them?

Many people who believe in detox steer clear of products altogether, protecting their systems from toxic overload simply by eating well and living cleanly. That usually means eating organic food (free of pesticides and genetic modification), avoiding polluted areas, and living where the air is cleaner. For other ideas, the website detox-guide.com is a good online source for all things detox. You might also want to look at detoxreviews.com, a site that reviews the hundreds of detox products on the market, from the Colonix & Toxinout Programs to the Intestinal Drawing Formula. And as far as not eating goes, *The Miracle of Fasting*, by Patricia Bragg and Paul C. Bragg, is a favorite book among aficionados, including Phil.

Eating Dirt

PATRICIA BURKE

Y ears ago, when Patricia Burke's sister introduced her British
fiancé to her family, they were stunned by his overwhelming
odor. Due in part to overactive central heating and perhaps
nervousness, the smell also derived from the man's infrequent
showers, born of his belief that Americans overbathed, thus killing off
mountains of good bacteria on their skin.

Patricia agreed with the fiancé: Her secret to good health is letting
her body maintain an adequate level of helpful bacteria—in her case,
inside her body.

A native New Yorker, Patricia came by her philosophy while visiting
her grandfather's prize-winning vegetable garden in northern Westchester
County, where he grew almost all the family's fresh food during the
summers: peas, beans, squash, beets, rhubarb, lettuce, and tomatoes.

She remembers grabbing fat, red tomatoes, hot from the sun, dipping them lightly in the icy-cold swimming pool, and shoving them into her mouth: "It was like eating a perfect day, one that smelled of the earth."

Also in the garden were peas, which she would open and eat off the vine. "They smelled delicious," she recalls, "and tasted like candy." Like the peas, all the vegetables were eaten straight from the garden, without much rinsing and with no consequences.

And while the house in which she grew up was neat and clean, mice and bugs sometimes visited. No one cared. To this day, mice don't bother her. Throughout her life, her habit has been to ignore dirt: "I drop food and I eat it. I don't care."

Patricia's philosophy was confirmed when a doctor explained to her the basis of vaccination: Injecting a bit of the disease you wish to prevent into a healthy person allows the body to build up an immunity to it. "I think exposing myself to a little bit of 'sick' allows my body to create its own defenses against passing germs, dirt, viruses, or whatever," she says.

At sixty-five, Patricia still eats vegetables straight from the garden after a desultory rinse, swallows food that's fallen on the floor, and doesn't wash her hands more than three or four times a day. That way, she feels she is "dosing" herself with all the microorganisms that can cause disease. She says the practice is why she is never sick.

Today, when she isn't at her job at a New York literary agency, she travels all over the world: drinking from rivers in South Africa, eating berries off bushes in Botswana, tasting mush in a village in Zimbabwe, sipping mare's milk in Mongolia, and munching on rice cakes in Chungking "that were kept in a drawer." Meanwhile, at home, her husband has threatened to put a REST IN PEACE sign on the food in their refrigerator.

The Facts on Eating Dirt

People in different parts of the world become ill and die in different ways. Infectious diseases such as pneumonia, malaria, and cholera account for the majority of deaths in the developing world. In the developed world, however, people more often suffer from a host of conditions epidemiologists classify as diseases of affluence, such as heart conditions and diabetes.

When Patricia doesn't worry about the bits of dirt that cling to her food or inhabit her environment, she is adhering to what is known as "the hygiene hypothesis," a theory about these diseases of affluence that reflects a paradigmatic shift in how medicine views the human immune system. Scientists have stopped regarding all bacteria, viruses, and fungi as unpleasant invaders with which we wage a pitched battle for territory in our bodies. Instead they have begun to view these microbes as symbiotes, or coinhabitants of our system. Considering that there are nearly ten to twenty times as many bacteria as human cells in our bodies, we are, in a sense, minorities within ourselves. Because of this fact, many medical professionals are beginning to believe that it's healthier for us to encourage, rather than stifle, their presence.

> "BE CAREFUL *about reading health books. You may die of a misprint.*"
> ~MARK TWAIN, AMERICAN WRITER

The shift in thinking began in 1989, when an English epidemiologist named David Strachan published a comprehensive study in the *British Medical Journal* on hay fever and eczema in children. Starting with a sample of more than seventeen thousand British children born during one week in 1958, Strachan interviewed them or their parents several times, even as late as twenty-three years later, in 1981, examining the resulting data in terms of different social and environmental factors. He found only one of these factors to be significant enough to suggest a causal relationship: family size. The greater the number of siblings the subject had, the lower the chance he or she had of developing either hay fever or eczema.

Strachan concluded that exposure to infections helps kids avoid allergies. "Over the past century, declining family size, improvements in household amenities, and higher standards of personal cleanliness have reduced opportunity for cross-infection in young families," he wrote.

In other words, increasing wealth, along with its demographic implications and resulting hygienic and cultural practices, helps explain

PICKING YOUR NOSE

◆

It's rare to see people pick their noses in public, but surveys have indicated that somewhere between 75 and 90 percent of Americans do so in private—some at least four times a day. It's a habit that people develop when young and that stays with them for the rest of their lives.

But is it harmless, or does it make you ill?

Possibly the latter. For the most part, cold viruses are passed into the body through the mucous membranes, most of which reside in your nose. If your fingers are contaminated through contact with an infected surface or person, sticking your fingers directly into your nose can cause an immediate transfer of that virus into your body. Furthermore, nature has placed hairs in your nose for a reason: They filter out tiny particles and some pollutants, preventing them from advancing farther into your system. When you pick your nose and pull out a hair, you're engaging in a form of friendly fire, plucking off a soldier in your immunity army. Now some enemy germ can venture past.

However, a second opinion: Dr. Friedrich Bischinger, a lung specialist based in Innsbruck, Austria, says picking your nose is actually beneficial because it helps clean out nasty particles that you can't blow out with a tissue. He even thinks it's a good idea to swallow what you pick, because the process strengthens the immune system by exposing it to invaders it needs to know more about (in case they show up en masse someday). Picking your nose and eating the results: You're an advocate of the hygiene hypothesis.

the rise in inflammatory and allergic diseases in developed countries over the last thirty years. Many of us aren't being exposed to enough of the germs that cause these ailments, so the body becomes hypersensitive not only to them but to microbes in general.

Very simply put, the human body has two ways of fighting off potentially harmful microbes: Th1-mediated immune response, and Th2-mediated immune response. Both of these immunological pathways block the harmful effects of certain pathogens by issuing microbe-fighting proteins called antibodies that cause inflammation and allergic symptoms

MORE DIRT ON DIRT

◆

It isn't just *eating* dirt that's good for you. Playing in it can be good for your health too, according to a 2009 study carried out by Northwestern University of more than 1,500 kids in the Philippines. The team discovered that the more pathogens children encountered outside before the age of two, the less inflammation found in their blood. The study suggests that early exposure to germs can reduce the risk of chronic inflammation later in life, thus reducing the risk of developing any number of serious conditions.

Likewise, scientists at the University of California–San Diego (UCSD) have found that the more bacteria you have crawling about the surface of your skin, the better you can combat inflammation. By studying mice and human cells, the UCSD team found that the bacteria can reduce inflammation after injury when they are present on the skin's surface. Apparently the microscopic bugs reduce an overactive immune response, which can lead to rashes, or cause cuts and bruises to become swollen and painful.

such as sniffling, sneezing, and rashes. The Th1 response also regulates the Th2 response, however, and therein lies the problem. If the Th1 response is not stimulated enough, the Th2 response goes haywire. When confronted with an allergen (say, tree pollen), the overly vigilant Th2 response acts a bit like a group of nervous soldiers firing their weapons all at once at a false alarm. Thus, allergic diseases like eczema, hay fever, and asthma are triggered by otherwise harmless microbes that nevertheless activate the body's immune response as though they were pathogens.

If it seems counterintuitive to say we should expose ourselves to the same bacteria, viruses, and other infectious organisms that can make us symptomatic, remember that our immune system evolved in an environment very different from today's. Many thousands of years ago, our ancestors were teeming with enough infectious creatures to require an all-out assault from the immune system to keep us alive. Our immune system is still calibrated to deal with a high level of exposure to these bugs, despite modern lifestyles. Unfortunately, the same medical advances that have allowed us to separate ourselves from the conditions under which we evolved have also altered the relationship between microbes and our immune system.

One of the first studies to show a concrete basis for the hygiene hypothesis confirmed the link between microorganisms and immune-response regulation. Researchers at the University of San Diego found that a harmless strain of *Staphylococcus* dampens the inflammation response to minor injuries. In a series of chemical calls and responses, the bacterium convinces the body's troops to chill out and stand down, thus avoiding unnecessary inflammation. *Staphylococcus,* by the way, is commonly found in dirt—a substance our ancestors probably ate a great deal of.

Still, no one is really calling for a return to prehistoric standards of hygiene. After all, antimicrobial sanitary products, advances in food hygiene, and evolving standards of cleanliness all have contributed to our ever increasing life expectancy. However, the hygiene hypothesis suggests that complete sterility is not necessarily always healthful and that the path to increasing health exists somewhere between the squalor of our ancestral environment and the hypercleanliness of the developed world.

Like most medical hypotheses, the hygiene one has flaws. For example, a better predictor of some conditions, such as asthma, is genetics: If both your parents have it, you're 60 percent more likely than others to have it as well. The hypothesis also has potential to do harm. One of its leading experts, Dr. Gerald Callahan, who studies bacteria and infectious diseases at Colorado State University, warns that we shouldn't simply start eating dirt. Except for friendly bacteria, there is much to avoid in modern soil: untreated human waste, heavy metals, fertilizers, and all the toxic agents associated with population density, industry, and modern agriculture.

Still, the fact remains that bacteria and our bodies exist in a symbiotic relationship in which their presence helps our systems remain healthy and balanced. In turn, we provide them a setting in which they can flourish: "Good" germs can improve your metabolism, enhance your immunity, and reduce inflammation in the body.

Share in the Secret

How can we give our children strong immune systems without the neighbors calling child services? While some scientists believe that a close relationship with animals (like those found on a farm) is the key to raising robust children, others feel the research remains inconclusive. Still, multiple studies point to a link between hookworm infection and a strong resistance to allergies, with one American-owned company in Mexico offering "inoculations" (intentional infections) for $3,900 a shot. Despite the promising evidence, it's important to remember that even if hookworms do block allergies, they are also one of the primary causes of malnutrition in the developing world.

As is often the case, the truth of the hygiene hypothesis probably lies somewhere in the middle of the road, as summed up by Marc McMorris, MD, a pediatric allergist at the University of Michigan Health System. He advises parents to "let kids be kids. If something like H1N1 is in the air, it's a good idea to wash your hands and take appropriate precautions. But you don't need to isolate your children from the world." This means you should keep immunizing them, but let them go outside, get dirty, and come in contact with Mother Nature.

So follow Dr. Callahan's advice: Don't eat a bowl of dirt for breakfast. But you might want to cease stressing so much about cleanliness. Instead, find a healthy compromise between sterility and filth. Rather than scrub your foods into unconsciousness, just give them a quick rinse. Don't fixate on what the cat drags in or on the dust balls beneath the bed. Be prudent without being obsessive. Moderation in all germs.

That said, each person's system has a different reaction to microorganisms. Someone with a history of inviting germs into her body will react differently to microorganisms than someone who has seldom been exposed to them. What works for Patricia may not work for you.

Friends

SYDNEY KLING

ydney Kling takes friendship seriously. On June 1, 2007, she began writing down the name of one person she spoke to each day—with the goal of never repeating a name. It began as a game to see how many different people she met during a specified period of time—as well as a test of how long she could do it and of how many friends she could make in the process.

For the first couple of months, the task was easy because she talked mainly to her current friends. But she also realized that if she paid attention, more often than not she could find new people with whom to get acquainted, gathering the names of a waitress, a bartender, a salesclerk, the person sitting beside her in church, a neighbor out walking her dog, and so on. As long as these personal encounters led to a brief conversation, she could count them. She also began adding her e-mail contacts to the list if more than one e-mail had been exchanged. Two years later, she had collected more than 750 names.

Sydney has mentioned this practice to only a few people because she knows it sounds somewhat compulsive. But she is determined to keep making friends for the rest of her life, because it's her secret to health.

Born seventy-five years ago on a small farm in southwest Minnesota, Sydney has called many different places home. Her parents moved repeatedly when she was young; after relocating to San Francisco to earn a bachelor's degree in nursing (followed later by a master's in counseling), she married and moved to Baton Rouge, Louisiana. Her husband subsequently took a job as a salesman, and the couple moved from town to town across the Midwest.

Sydney's career also placed her in a variety of different settings and hospitals, as she migrated from specialty to specialty and position to position—labor and delivery, orthopedics, night supervisor, coronary-care specialist. Eventually she took up teaching, spending two decades working for the state of Illinois, during which time she set up newborn screening and genetic counseling programs, among other things.

After she retired, she joined the Peace Corps and lived for two years in South Africa, where she was a home volunteer for patients with HIV. She later participated in volunteer programs in Greece, the Ukraine, China, and Costa Rica.

Despite switching locales and undergoing a painful divorce, Sydney, who now lives in Springfield, Illinois, recalls no illnesses; her four stays in the hospital were for the births of her four children. She insisted on natural childbirth, unusual in the 1940s and '50s. "I knew those doctors," she says. "I wasn't about to let them put me to sleep."

She believes what's kept her healthy through all the moves and jobs is her intense social networking, which started when she was three years old. "When I was young, there were a dozen kids in my class. I lived in town, and the rest of the girls lived on farms. The boys lived in the town, however, so every day I'd walk to school with three or four of them. They

FRIENDSHIP AND GENDER

The impetus for friendships among women—but not men—may be more biological in origin than previously thought. According to a recent UCLA study published in *Psychology Today*, cultivating friendships is the primary method women use to cope with stress. When confronted with difficult situations, the study found that men succumbed to the fight-or-flight response, but women employed a "tend and befriend" pattern—tending to children, befriending other females.

In explaining the differing behavior patterns, the UCLA team pointed to the hormone oxytocin, which has been studied primarily for its role in childbirth but is also secreted by both men and women in response to stress. Higher oxytocin levels in animals have been linked to maternalism and affiliation. The female hormone estrogen seems to enhance this response. The male hormone testosterone, on the other hand, squelches production of oxytocin. Along this line of thinking, women are more likely to seek out friendships because, when they engage fully in tending or befriending, their bodies release still *more* oxytocin, countering the effects of stress.

treated me like one of them. I would tell them which girl was nice, which girls wore falsies."

Having studied genetics, Sydney suspects she inherited a strong immune system but wonders if she also inherited a genetic disposition for sociability. Sociability, she claims, increases self-esteem, which, in turn, supports the immune system. "When my husband left me, I felt terrible. Having friends brought my self-esteem back. Not just through their help, but through my helping them: Having people rely on you is important."

The Facts on Friends

"You've got to have friends," goes the song. Sounds obvious, except for the fact that many people don't.

The common complaint about modern life—"I can't make any friends"—has been studied extensively, and multiple theories explain the phenomenon. Sociologists like the late Max Lerner attribute the phenomenon to the breakdown of community within American society. Through the last half of the twentieth century, the migration of people from small towns to cities and the subsequent rise of the suburb have fragmented Americans' lives into many separate compartments—spaces in which people seldom interact on more than a purely superficial level.

"IN THE FUTURE *we'll all have fifteen minutes of fame and fifteen minutes of healthcare.*"

~NICOLE HOLLANDER, AMERICAN CARTOONIST

In his classic work *The Great Good Place,* urban sociologist Ray Oldenburg identified the three places that play the most significant roles in our lives. The first is the house. Used as a retreat from the outside world, its inherent purpose serves to isolate rather than integrate us.

The second place is work, where we meet many people but make few friends, due to the fact that everyone actually lives elsewhere—and heads there immediately after work. Moreover, the workplace is restricted by policies that hamper our ability to interact freely.

The third place is the informal public gathering spot. In England, it's the pub; in France, the café; in Italy, the piazza, and so on. Modern-day America does not have an equivalent, although to some degree the Internet has become the new watering hole. But studies show that face-to-face connections tend to be stronger than online ones, because it's easier to establish intimacy, trust, and reciprocity while interacting without the mediation of a keyboard.

Just as opportunities to make friends have been waning, studies about its health benefits have been waxing. Having friends can reduce stress and anxiety: Numerous studies have shown that having social support decreases the heart-racing, blood pressure–boosting human stress response. A 2009 article in the *Journal of the National Medical Association,* for example, found that social support can relieve stress;

studies have also shown that people with close support from friends and family have fewer inflammatory chemicals in their blood.

Similarly, university researchers at Ohio State and Pittsburgh's Carnegie Mellon University have demonstrated that people who report having strong social support have more robust immune systems and are less likely to succumb to infectious disease. Moreover, a ten-year Australian study estimated that older people with a large circle of friends were 22 percent less likely to die during the study period than those with fewer friends.

The presence—or absence—of friends cuts across a spectrum of possible conditions. A 2008 Harvard study showed that strong social ties could "[protect] against memory loss and other cognitive disorders," and a 2006 study published in the *Journal of Clinical Oncology* showed that "socially isolated women had an elevated risk of mortality after a diagnosis of breast cancer, likely because of a lack of access to care, specifically beneficial caregiving from friends, relatives, and adult children."

Other studies on the absence of friends support the notion of their importance to health. A recent Swedish study of middle-aged men found that having few or no close friends increases the risk of having a first-time heart attack by about 50 percent. A 2002 Harvard School of Public Health study of more than 28,000 men revealed that those without strong social ties were nearly 20 percent more likely to die within a decade. And a 2009 study in Buffalo, New York, found that those with the fewest social ties were the most likely to suffer from heart disease, anxiety, and depression.

Recently researchers have been looking at the effects of friendship from a different angle: behavior. Using data from the Framingham Heart Study—one of the longest-lasting and most influential health studies ever conducted, run under the direction of the National Heart, Lung and Blood Institute (NHLBI)—social scientists Nicholas Christakis and James Fowler discovered that friends have a more powerful effect on one another than scientists had previously thought.

ALONE AGAIN

◆

Just as friendship is contagious, so is loneliness. According to research published in the *Journal of Personality and Social Psychology* in 2009, data from the Framingham Heart Study show that if someone in your social network is lonely, you yourself are 52 percent more likely to be lonely as well. If the degree of separation is two (a friend of a friend), you are 25 percent more likely to be lonely.

According to the study, loneliness spreads much more easily among women than among men—although this fact might be affected by the fact that women are more willing to admit to loneliness than men, who tend to be less likely to confess aloud any weakness.

For example, they noticed that if one person became obese, his or her friends were 57 percent more likely to become obese as well. Similarly, being around smokers was more likely to make a nonsmoker take up the habit, while people surrounded by happy people were more likely to be happy too. Other studies have shown that people are more likely to exercise, remember medical appointments, and talk to someone when they feel down if they have friends.

Why does friendship convey so many benefits beyond curing loneliness? Perhaps it's simply that being around healthy people with healthy habits encourages us to accompany them in their salubrious activities or to emulate them. But friendship is no panacea. For instance, as mentioned in the introduction, being in close proximity to friends may spread colds. While for many years doctors believed that people were more likely to catch a cold in winter's chill (and yes, that's the origin of the term *cold*), it turns out that low temperatures matter less than spending more time indoors surrounded by other people's germs. This theory adds weight to the observation that the healthier the people around you are, the more likely it is that you, too, will stay healthy.

Share in the Secret

Online communities like Facebook make it seemingly easy to cultivate friends. But are Facebook friends real friends? A survey conducted by researchers at Sheffield Hallam University in the U.K. found that the average number of friends on social networks was 150. Of those, 5 were "core" friends, the rest, cyber acquaintances.

Twenty-three-hundred years before Facebook, the philosopher Aristotle wrote, "A friend is a single soul dwelling in two bodies." He further defined friendship as existing between "those who desire the good of their friends for the friends' sake . . . because each loves the other for what he is, and not for any incidental quality."

Whatever your definition of a friend, there is no simple way to make one. Thousands of how-to books have been written on the subject, and if any one of them had been completely accurate, the rest of them wouldn't have been published.

Being proactive, however, is a good start. Here are tips from business consultant Tim Sanders, the author of several bestselling books on relationship building, including *Love is the Killer App*.

1. **Start with your current social situation** Maybe you already have the potential to make new friends right now. Are you getting to know everyone at work? At the club or church? On the bus or the train? For the next few weeks, strike up at least two conversations every day with someone whom you haven't talked to before.

2. **Listen more than you speak.** To paraphrase Dale Carnegie, author of the immense bestseller How to Win Friends and Influence People, you'll accomplish more in the next few months developing a sincere interest in two people than you'll accomplish in the next few months trying to get two people interested in you. Resist the temptation to make points or interrupt when someone says something that triggers a thought. The more airtime you give someone, the more generous he or she will be with personal details.

3. **Connect at the passion level.** People love to talk about their personal passions more than work or even family. Ask someone, "What are you going to do this weekend?" instead of "What do you do for a living?" My research tells me that you have a 70 percent chance of finding a loose tie between one of your new acquaintance's passions and one of your own.

4. **Be helpful, especially when others voice a need.** Being helpful is the best way to trigger the social norm of reciprocity, so others want to help you back. Mutual value is the foundation of a friendship. Listen for opportunities to make a difference or lend support, and never ask for repayment.

5. **Treat feelings as facts.** When people voice their emotions, they usually just want to be heard, especially when they are sad. When you treat these feelings as legitimate, you give the other person a powerful sense of validation, which can often alleviate his or her suffering. This is also true of positive emotions, such as excitement or joy. Respond with enthusiasm and reinforce your friend's happiness.

6. **Stay in touch.** Many friendships dissolve over time as we fail to keep in high contact (by face or phone). We get busy, we relegate the relationship to digital venues (e-mail, Facebook), and soon our friends are former friends. Don't expect a great experience in the past to be powerful enough to keep a friendship alive in the future.

7. **Limit your complaints.** Your tone can determine how often others want to converse with you. If you come across as a Needy Nancy or Whiny Will, you'll get screened out. This doesn't mean you can't talk about real and difficult issues, but try to balance the bad in your life with the good.

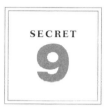

SECRET

9

Garlic

SUSAN SEIDEMAN BROWN

Fifty-one-year-old Susan Brown, who has lived most of her life near Philadelphia, Pennsylvania, is preparing to move off the grid. She and her thirty-four-year-old boyfriend have decided that they've had enough of the world as it is. They intend to stop paying for electricity and water, take care of their own sewage, and rely on solar and wind power and a wood-burning stove. Their goal is to avoid harming the environment while detaching themselves from a political and social system they feel has grown too large and unwieldy.

To do this, Susan's boyfriend will build a log cabin somewhere in the Northeast, then make a living building them for other people. Susan will continue in her present career as a shiatsu massage therapist. (Previously, she ran a health food store, until she decided she couldn't simultaneously manage the business and raise her two children.) "I can't think of anything we will miss," she says. "We both like a simple life."

However simple their new life, garlic will be a part of it.

Susan was exposed to the idea that food was important when she was young. Her mother is a "vegan with a mission—she makes sourpuss faces at anyone who eats anything else." Seventy-four (and healthy), Susan's mother now runs an alternative health center in Delaware.

Susan herself got into thinking about food when she was fifteen and suffering from bad mood swings, irritability, and exhaustion. She stopped eating sugars and drinking sodas—and felt better. Some years later, while having terrible stomachaches, she determined that the cause was a gall-bladder issue and stopped eating creamy, rich, and fried foods. Again she felt better.

She also came down with the flu every year. Then her boyfriend told her about garlic.

"He said that garlic cures everything. So one night, when I thought I was getting sick, I cut off a clove of raw garlic, let it dissolve in my mouth, and the cold was gone. Now, anytime I think I'm getting sick, I start with the garlic three times a day, and within twenty-four hours, I feel fine."

Susan also takes garlic "preventatively." She cooks with it each day, putting it in every dinner, which tends to include vegetables, onions, and some kind of starch, such as rice or pasta. And she squeezes raw garlic on top of the dish as well.

Although some people notice that garlic gives them body odor or bad breath, she denies it. "If you have kids, you know they'd be the first to tell you. And mine don't." Nor do her outspoken massage clients, who experience her breath often, and close up.

The Facts on Garlic

A member of the lily, or Allium, family, which also includes onions, leeks, and chives, garlic, aka the stinking rose, is first known to have been cultivated in central Asia in the Neolithic era. Though historians continue to debate its primary function in ancient times, we know it was used to flavor food and for medicinal purposes.

Many early civilizations used garlic for the latter. Tablets dating from 3000 B.C. show that the Assyrians and Sumerians employed garlic to treat fevers, inflammation, and injuries. Clay sculptures of garlic bulbs and paintings of garlic dating to about 3200 B.C. have been found in Egyptian tombs, as well as a papyrus from 1500 B.C. recommending garlic as a cure for more than twenty medical conditions. The pyramid builders fed it to laborers to increase their strength (a fact inscribed on the Great Pyramid of Cheops), and the only Egyptian slave revolt was triggered by a lack of garlic (an overflowing Nile had destroyed that year's crop).

The Israelites also used garlic, before and after leaving Egypt: In the Mishnah, a collection of Jewish traditions incorporated into the Talmud, ancient Hebrew writers call themselves "the garlic eaters," and in Numbers 11:5, Jews traveling to the Promised Land bemoan garlic's absence.

Roman naturalist Pliny the Elder (23–79 A.D.) recommended it to repel serpents, soothe animal bites and toothache, and as an aphrodisiac. Hippocrates thought garlic could cure cancer. In the Middle Ages, the German nun Saint Hildegard of Bingen recommended garlic to heal the sick, and in 1665 the London College of Physicians recommended garlic to treat the great plague.

By the nineteenth century, researchers investigating the medicinal effects of garlic were finding corroboration. In 1858, for example, Louis Pasteur discovered that garlic kills bacteria: One milliliter of raw garlic juice was as effective as 60 milligrams of penicillin.

Public awareness about the benefits of garlic has been increasing—which helps explain why garlic is now second only to echinacea (see page 92) in sales of herbal supplements. The primary focus of much of the enormous quantity of favorable research has been cardiovascular benefits. For example, India's Tagore Medical College performed a study showing that test subjects who consumed garlic experienced a drop in blood pressure of about 10 percent; a Czech study discovered that garlic supplements lessened cholesterol accumulation on animals' vascular walls.

Garlic has also been shown to reduce blood pressure and triglyceride and cholesterol levels and to increase the production of nitric oxide in the lining of the blood vessel walls, which relaxes them, allowing blood and nutrients to flow more easily. And, it can inhibit coronary artery calcification and aid in the prevention of atherosclerotic plaque formation. (Atherosclerosis is a form of arteriosclerosis, or degenerative changes of arteries; plaque is a fatty substance that forms deposits on the inner lining of arterial walls.)

Other studies show that garlic can act as a powerful antioxidant and an antibiotic, as at least one study has shown that garlic fights off a very dangerous strain of *Staphylococcus,* the bug that causes staph infections. And yes, as Susan experienced, garlic is helpful in the battle against the common cold—at least, so found a 2007 study from the Garlic Centre in East Sussex, England. Likewise, researchers at the University of Western Australia discovered that people taking garlic reduced by more than half the number of days they were sick. They also found a dramatic reduction in the number of colds caught.

However, for all the goods news, there have been a few setbacks to garlic's reputation. Some studies were unable to show any efficacy in treating various conditions, and there is also the question of just how *much* it helps. A 2007 study by the National Center for Complementary and Alternative Medicine, for example, raised questions about the cholesterol-reducing and cardiological benefits of garlic, documented in previous reports, concluding that garlic has no impact on LDL cholesterol levels.

It's also possible to take too much garlic or to take it at the wrong time. For hemophiliacs and others with blood-clotting problems, garlic can cause problems. Used medicinally—that is, in high doses—garlic has a thinning effect on the blood, which can be dangerous for these patients. Also, if garlic is applied externally, its caustic oils can sometimes irritate the skin.

Some people suffer from allergies to plants in the Allium family. Symptoms can include irritable bowels, diarrhea, mouth and throat ulcerations, nausea, breathing difficulties, and, in rare cases, anaphylaxis (shock). Even if garlic is present in a very small amount, it can lead to an allergic reaction in sensitive individuals.

GARLIC AND THE UNDEAD

The belief that garlic can ward off vampires flourished in Romania, home of Vlad the Impaler, aka Prince Dracula. Whenever medieval Romanians feared a corpse might become undead, they'd stuff garlic into its orifices and smear the body with rendered fat, oil, and more garlic.

Oddly, it wasn't just Romania where this custom was common. According to British vampire expert Montague Summers, the Chinese and Malaysians rubbed their children's foreheads with garlic to protect them from vampires; in the West Indies, garlic is used to protect against the evil practices of witches and sorcerers.

As to *why* garlic was thus used, no one seems to know, although French occult expert Robert Ambelain wrote that it may have originated with Carpathian shepherds who hired alchemists to protect their sheep from vampires. The alchemists complied by burning arsenic, which smells like garlic, until the resourceful and frugal shepherds fired the alchemists and began using actual garlic, which was much cheaper.

More recently, scientists have taken a look at the connection between garlic and bloodsuckers. No experiments with actual vampires have been conducted, but a number of tests involving garlic and blood have shown that garlic, when ingested, enters the bloodstream far less adulterated than average food. When viruses come across it in a creature's veins, they flee. So garlic can repel blood-borne viruses. Viruses. Vampires. Not so different.

Conversely, two scientists at the University of Bergen in Norway discovered that garlic might have an unwanted effect. Substituting for vampires in their informal study were bloodsucking leeches that, when given a choice between garlic-smeared and clean flesh, chose the garlicky flesh two times out of three. The garlic-loving hermaphroditic annelids also attached themselves and set to sucking the flesh thirty-five seconds faster than the garlic-avoiding ones.

Finally, garlic can interact with prescription medications, so if you intend to add large amounts of garlic to your diet, as is often the case, talk to your doctor first.

Share in the Secret

Garlic can be ingested in many ways. Some people cook it and some eat it raw—which is fine if you can abide the taste as well as the resulting pungent breath that many claim lingers on and on. (Current research doesn't indicate whether one form is more healthful than the other.)

Garlic is processed into many liquid forms, such as teas and syrups. It also is available in pill form. Many garlic experts disparage the pills, however, claiming that the process of making them may destroy the flower's power. For example, garlic researcher Dr. David Kraus of the University of Alabama at Birmingham says that much of garlic's medicinal value is related to its odor. When a compound in garlic called allinin is converted to allicin (as when a bulb is crushed or damaged), garlic gives off hydrogen sulfide, its gassy smell. He warns against odorless supplements, saying that if the release of hydrogen sulfide is sacrificed, you won't be getting garlic's full benefits.

"AMERICA'S HEALTH care system is neither healthy, caring, nor a system."

~WALTER CRONKITE, AMERICAN BROADCASTER

Others point out that allicin isn't present in raw garlic. Instead, it forms in your mouth within seconds as you eat it, when an enzyme known as allinase turns allinin into allicin. If you take a garlic pill, the stomach's acidic environment can prevent the necessary conversion from taking place.

If you do decide to eat garlic, the most potent form is fresh. Store it in a loosely covered container away from heat and sunlight. It need not be refrigerated, and will keep for up to two months.

Do not store garlic in oil at room temperature, however. Such mixtures provide the perfect conditions for producing dangerous botulism, regardless of whether the garlic is fresh or has been roasted first.

A DASH OF ZUG

❖

Susan Brown's favorite way to add garlic to her diet is via a spread she uses on toast or tosses into a stir fry or pasta dish. She likes to make more than she needs and freeze some for later. That way, there's always a little zug on hand.

2 cups parsley (or cilantro)

4 cloves garlic

3 hot peppers, diced

½ small onion, coarsely chopped

½ mango, diced

⅓ cup olive oil

Salt and black pepper to taste

Blend ingredients together until well mixed.

YIELD: *About 1 cup*

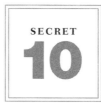

Germ Avoidance

RACHEL HILL

When Rachel Hill decides to take her horse for a long ride, she plans the journey months in advance. An October ride means a January start to prepare her horse for the snowy ride in Canada's extreme winter weather. By spring she'll be taking the horse for extended rides; by summer, making eight-mile treks before work.

Then she has to start preparing her gear as well as her horse's—plus focus on the registration, vetting, meal-planning, as well as taking care of the horse's feed and electrolytes, and buying the T-shirts that say things such as RIDE TILL YOU PUKE.

And that's what she does, now and then, because Rachel's hobby is endurance riding. The sport takes her and her horse many dozens of miles over steep hills, across rushing rivers, and atop soft sand, shale, and whatever else nature serves up. Just being able to finish the ride is the prize; doing so may mean trekking fifty miles or more in a single day. Her eventual goal: to finish a hundred-miler.

Rachel, who grew up in rural northeastern Ontario, is an environmental consultant working on diverse projects, from environment assessments and renewable energy programs to dam developments and wind farms. Her career involves spending a great deal of time outdoors in harsh climates.

Nonetheless, Rachel rarely gets sick. The last time was about nine years ago, when the Norwalk virus swept through town—an epidemic so severe that senior citizens' homes were closed and visitors weren't allowed at local hospitals.

That's when Rachel stopped using the pen at her local Fort Frances, Ontario, grocery store.

One day while waiting to sign for her purchases, Rachel noticed that everyone around her was sniffling and coughing, then handling the pen. After that, she caught the flu. So she decided to avoid unnecessary human contact.

> "I AM LIKE A DETECTIVE *about any room in which I must live or work.... I will not chance a serious illness just because I'm told that spraying is 'customary.' Of course bugs can be annoying, but I prefer to take my chances with them, if spraying of deadly chemicals into the air I breathe is the only alternative."*
>
> —GLORIA SWANSON, AMERICAN FILM STAR

Now she'll take a shopping cart that's been left standing out in the heat or cold rather than one recently used by people. Just to be sure, she'll swab it with sanitizer she carries in her purse. She also takes extra care in public restrooms: After washing her hands, she'll choose a paper towel over a blow dryer because air dryers aren't thoroughly efficient, because Rachel feels damp hands can pick up bugs. She then uses the paper to grasp the door handle when she exits.

In shopping centers, she avoids using hand rails or keeps her gloves on. She minimizes visits to food courts, but if she must partake, she skips the cold salad bar and sticks with hot, cooked dishes.

When possible, Rachel takes the stairs instead of riding an elevator; if she hears someone sneeze in a confined space, she automatically holds her breath "in hopes that the germs whiz by me by the time I have to breathe again."

However, she's not at all worried by nonhuman germs: "I touch animals constantly and ingest animals' dirt all the time—when has someone picked up a stomach flu from a dog? The bad stuff you're going to pick up is from a person."

Therefore, she washes her hands often and avoids touching her face after human contact. She recalls, "One winter not long ago I was flying helicopter moose surveys and the helicopter landed to pick me up. As the pilot walked over, he was blowing his nose, and then held out a hand for me to shake. I shook it, but thought about my contaminated hand all day; I even ate my lunch with the 'good' hand."

The Facts on Germ Avoidance

The hygiene hypothesis (see page 50) suggests that humans need more, not less, contact with microorganisms. People like Rachel Hill are fine with that, as long as the germs come from a dirty tomato and not from people infected with a cold.

Germs are any kind of microorganism that causes illness in their host. Also called pathogens, they comprise an unpleasant family of infinitesimally small creatures divided into four main groups: bacteria, viruses, fungi, and protozoa.

Bacteria give us, among other things, strep throats and pneumonia; viruses are responsible for smallpox and AIDS; fungi cause athlete's foot; and protozoa provoke intestinal infections.

Before humans knew about the existence of germs, they deemed spirits, demons, unusual weather patterns, and mysterious bodily fluids responsible for illness. Infections were treated by bleeding, and mental illness might require that a hole be drilled in your skull. No one was safe from these interventions. As mentioned in the introduction, when George Washington came down with a respiratory infection in 1799, the best doctors in America gathered at his bedside and decided to treat him

ZOONOSES

◆

Rachel doesn't obsess over animals' germs, but some of them can be dangerous. Within the animal kingdom are a substantial number of zoonoses, or diseases that can be passed from animals to humans, and they aren't necessarily the ones that people fear most. Rabies, anthrax, swine flu, bird flu, and the plague are all well-documented zoonoses. Fortunately for us, they rarely make the jump from four legs to two: For instance, although still common in developing countries, rabies is relatively rare in the first world.

More important in terms of frequency are a group of less potent diseases that can still cause serious damage to humans. Toxoplasmosis, which comes from handling cat feces or eating undercooked meat, can cause a month of flulike symptoms and even kill the fetuses of pregnant women. Salmonella, contracted from reptiles and amphibians, causes diarrhea, which can be dangerous to children and people with suppressed immune systems. Giardia comes from drinking water infected by animal feces or eating underwashed fruit or vegetables. Though not lethal, it is another diarrhea causer and occurs frequently among campers and hikers. Another common zoonosis is cat-scratch fever, which infects as many as twenty thousand Americans every year with flulike symptoms. It may not be the plague, but it's a disease, like many zoonoses, that can easily be avoided by handling animals carefully and always washing your hands afterward.

by removing eighty ounces of blood from his body in a single day. The draining weakened him considerably, hastening his death.

Because these older treatments had a limited success rate, medical researchers kept working, and slowly, over centuries, the germ theory of disease advanced. In the fourteenth century, Arab doctors hypothesized that the Black Death was caused by minute contagious particles. Several centuries later, the Italian scientist Agostini Bassi first postulated a role for germs while studying an epidemic among silkworms. And, as also discussed in the introduction, germ-theory pioneer Ignaz Semmelweis realized in the mid-1800s that when hospital staff washed their hands

MYSOPHOBIA

◆

Avoidance of germs is sensible. But when it moves from a precautionary measure to an obsession, you've come down with mysophobia, the excessive fear of uncleanliness and germs. The term was first coined in 1879 by neurologist and Surgeon General of the U.S. Army William Alexander Hammond, who believed that the condition was a symptom of obsessive compulsive disorder (OCD) that was centered on repeated washing of the hands. However, doctors now debate whether mysophobia is always part of OCD, or if it also occurs as a disorder in itself.

What is clear is that the condition has been exhibited by many eccentric characters. For example, Nikola Tesla, the scientist responsible for fluorescent lighting, the alternating current electrical supply system, and the Tesla coil (among many other inventions), did not like to shake hands and, it was said, required eighteen napkins to get through a meal. He even developed a "bath" that would clean

before operating on patients, complications, such as puerperal fever, diminished. The medical profession wasn't ready to listen, even though scientists throughout Europe had been peering at tiny creatures under a microscope (perfected by the Dutchman Anton Van Leeuwenhoek, one of the fathers of microbiology) since the seventeenth century. Their work over the next two hundred years led them to develop theories on the role of microorganisms in causing illness. They reasoned that if they could prove a single cause for most illnesses, then a rigorous and scientific approach to fighting disease could be developed.

The best known of these scientists was Louis Pasteur, who in the 1850s and 1860s advanced the concept that mold and other growths on food and in homes did not in fact spring up out of nowhere (a concept known as spontaneous generation), but rather were produced by microorganisms. From this understanding, Pasteur went on to develop the technique of pasteurization, the process of heating fluid to kill the microorganisms within.

germs from the body using nothing but electrical current.

A more famous case is that of the aviator, movie producer, and one-time world's richest man, Howard Hughes, who became obsessively mysophobic as he grew older. A posthumous study in the *Monitor on Psychology* revealed someone who spent a great deal of time lying naked in darkened hotel rooms, wore tissue boxes on his feet, and burned his clothes if he came into close contact with a sick person.

Other mysophobes have included the pianist Glen Gould, who sometimes performed in a coat and scarf and disliked human contact; artist Andy Warhol, whose fear of germs and hospitals was legendary; and TV personality Howie Mandel, who fist-bumps contestants on his show, *Deal or No Deal,* to avoid shaking hands.

As some psychologists believe mysophobia in America is increasing due to wider knowledge of germs and diseases, it's wise to remember the words of English writer Gilbert Chesterton: "Man does not live by soap alone; and hygiene, or even health, is not much good unless you can take a healthy view of it or, better still, feel a healthy indifference to it."

Unlike many of the scientific breakthroughs of the nineteenth century, germ theory has not been called into question in modern times; rather, it has been affirmed and further refined. Now-common public health practices, including vaccination and the use of antibiotics, were instituted as a result of germ theory. Few other discoveries can claim to have saved more lives.

But just because we know about germs doesn't mean we can always defeat them. We're coming in contact with them constantly, and each one of us is an enormous depository of germs. That means that on the bus, in the classroom, in the boardroom, or at the ballgame, we are swapping one another's germs. Billions of them.

Infectious diseases kill more people around the world than any other cause. And in fact, 80 percent of all infections are said to be spread via touch, which is not so surprising when you realize that humans carry between 2 million and 10 million living bacteria between their fingertips and elbows—a number that increases

THE LIFE OF A GERM

How long does a germ live outside a human being? No one is quite sure. It depends on where it lands, which type it is, the surrounding temperature and humidity levels, and many other factors. Recent experiments with differing cold and flu germs have shown survival times that range from a few minutes to more than two days.

In general, it seems as though these germs last longer on hard surfaces, such as steel, glass, and plastic. They don't tend to thrive as well on cloth and fabrics.

But again, it's a matter of debate. According to Dr. Kent Sepkowitz, director of hospital infection control at Memorial Sloan-Kettering Cancer Center and professor of medicine at the Weill Medical College of Cornell University, the answer is probably "hours—not minutes, not days, and not weeks."

He continues: "The more confusing issue is that 'surviving' on an object such as a doorknob is not the same as being transmissible. In other words, if you put a quantity of cold virus on a doorknob and came back every hour to see how long you could successfully get it to grow in a culture, you would get a quantifiable answer. But whether the ability to be grown in culture is equivalent to being readily transmissible in nature is unknown." Still, most experts agree that it makes sense to wash your hands after any known contact with a contaminated surface.

every time we sneeze or cough into our hands, use the bathroom, or touch foreign objects.

The CDC estimates that 164 million school days are lost to illness each year. Although not all of these absences are caused by germs, a study of 305 schoolchildren conducted in Detroit schools showed that many illnesses were passed from one person to another. The study found that those kids who washed their hands four times a day had 24 percent fewer sick days caused by respiratory illness and 51 percent fewer days lost due to stomach upset than kids who didn't wash as frequently.

Germs are great independent travelers, too, jumping from human hands to tables, doorknobs, or keyboards, then back to human hands and into mouths or eyes, where they can infect a host. The CDC notes that some viruses and bacteria can survive for two hours or more on tables, doorknobs, and desks, just waiting to be picked up by unsuspecting people.

And they aren't always lurking where you might think. Contrary to popular belief, the most germ-infested area of the house isn't the bathroom. It's the kitchen. The most contaminated sites are the ones that remain damp, like the sink, refrigerator, and garbage can. At the office, telephone receivers probably harbor more germs than any other surface including the toilet bowl; elevator buttons and keyboards are a close second.

Still, although germ theory has been around for a century and a half, we don't understand it. Some people are clearly more susceptible to germs than others, and no one knows why. Some germs are more powerful than others, and that, too, is a mystery. Furthermore, some of what seems to be intuitively true isn't. For example, although washing your hands seems like a good way to avoid taking germs into your system, being *too* clean can give rise to *more* pathogens. Skin is a natural protection against germs, but washing it too often can throw off its water content, humidity, pH, intracellular lipids, and shedding rate, making it less able to do its job.

Given this fact, in 2001 the CDC recommended a reassessment of the "trend in both the general public and among health-care professionals toward more frequent washing with detergents, soaps, and antimicrobial ingredients... In light of the damage done to skin and resultant increased risk for harboring and transmitting infectious agents."

Share in the Secret

The only way to ensure that other people won't pass their germs along to you is to avoid other people entirely. Becoming a hermit, the ultimate mysophobe, is extreme, however, so it's better to look into two simple precautions emphasized by the CDC that can drastically reduce your chances of contracting other people's diseases.

First, and most obvious, avoid close contact with sick people. Germs can't infect things they aren't exposed to.

Second, avoid touching your nose, mouth, and eyes with your hand whenever possible: These are the points where pathogens enter your body, usually via your fingers and hands. Speaking of your hands, they tend to become dirty fairly quickly, so the single best way to prevent infection from other people's germs is to wash them before and after certain activities, including before cooking, after handling raw meat, after sneezing or coughing into your hand, and after using the bathroom.

Proper hand-washing isn't a quick dunk under the faucet, either. It's a five-step process, says the CDC:

1. Wet your hands with clean running water and apply soap. Use warm water if it is available.

2. Rub your hands together to make a lather and scrub all surfaces.

3. Continue rubbing your hands for fifteen to twenty seconds. If you don't have a timer nearby, this is about the time it would take to sing "Happy Birthday."

4. Rinse hands well under running water.

5. Dry your hands using a paper towel or air dryer. If possible, use your paper towel to turn off the faucet.

One popular trend in germ avoidance is the surgical mask worn in public places, as seen in many Asian cities and Mexico City during the 2009–10 H1N1 outbreak. However, many viruses are so small that they have no trouble passing through surgical masks, even through many of the specially designed masks known as N-95 respirators. On the other hand, a mask may make your fellow citizens question your mental well-being, giving you plenty of breathing room in public.

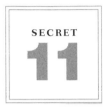

SECRET

11

Good Genes

MOUSSA MAMADOU

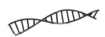

From 1974 to 1976, I was a Peace Corps volunteer (PCV) in the Republic of Niger, in West Africa. Niger, a francophone country in the Sahel, or the southern part of the Sahara, was languishing through one of the worst droughts in modern history; scores of people had starved to death. Niger was considered one of the most difficult posts in the Peace Corps. I'd wanted an assignment in the South Pacific or in southern Africa—not the parched desert—but like most PCVs, I fell in love with the country where I worked.

My job was to teach English to students who often spoke three or four languages already—French, along with local languages, such as Djerma, Hausa, or Fulani. My students were good with languages, and their English was passable, although they were never clear on my first name, which they pronounced "Jin." Usually, however, they called me Monsieur, Sir, or Stone ("Stun"). Then again, their names sounded equally odd to me: The front row of one class consisted of Moussa, Amadou, Mamadou, Mahaman, another Mamadou, another Moussa.

The second Moussa was a particularly friendly young man whose family lived in a nearby village. At a time when the country was barely surviving and the average income was well under one hundred dollars a year, Moussa often invited me to his home for dinner. There his family would serve up enough food for the two dozen or so friends and relatives, as well as me and perhaps another *anasara* (stranger).

Moussa was about twenty years old. His parents were probably about forty-five, although his father was maybe five years older than his mother. All four of his grandparents were alive and present; they must have been in their sixties or seventies. Four of Moussa's great-grandparents were also present; although I asked many times, no one ever told me how old they were, nor could I seem to find out where the other great-grandparents were. I was also told there was at least one great-great grandparent around, but again, she never materialized. (Sometimes I thought they might have been talking about a nonliving entity; when I brought it up, they just shrugged.)

Due to the ravages brought on by starvation, infectious diseases, and poor medical care, many Nigeriens were dying far too young; at the time, they had one of the lowest life expectancies in the world—forty-one years. But Moussa and his family were seldom ill and they lived longer lives than most people in developed countries. There was no difference between their diet and that of their friends, no difference in their exercise patterns (there wasn't a gym in the country, but people walked miles, often carrying heavy objects). There was only a difference in their health and longevity. When I asked them about it, all I got were more shrugs.

The Facts on Genetics

Why is it that some people (or entire families) always seem to be healthy—no matter what they do, how they act, or where they live? It's a question that's been asked for centuries. But one of the few questions that's been asked more than that one is actually related to it—and that question is "Where do babies come from?"

As is often the case, Hippocrates was among the first Westerners to offer an answer to the latter question. Children, he explained, are created from fluids distilled from the parents' bodily organs (lungs, heart, pancreas, and so on), and these fluids combine during sexual intercourse.

Aristotle later contributed his own theory: The male's seed is distilled from his blood, which contains his *pneuma*, or spirit. The woman's seed, contained in her menstrual blood, modifies this spirit. The resulting child's sex will depend on the temperature: If you want to conceive a boy, wait for a warm day; if a girl, seek a cooler encounter.

Over the centuries, scientists learned more about the details of reproduction but struggled to understand what determines human traits. Meanwhile, European animal breeders were developing ways to raise stronger, faster, and more docile animals. As Jim Endersby writes in his book *A Guinea Pig's History of Biology,* these efforts employed "a complex mixture of first-hand experience, classical learning, and folk myth" and represented the first, perhaps unwitting, steps toward a true understanding of the principles of inheritance.

Breeders and scientists finally began to take an interest in each other's ideas in the seventeenth century, and by the nineteenth century, the cross-pollination had produced the first generation of biologists formally investigating the mechanics of genetic heredity in plants and animals. Many of their early hypotheses were off-base, however, such as Sir Francis Galton's infamous theory of eugenics, which posited that the human race could be improved through selective breeding.

Then along came a monk and a pea. In 1865, the Austrian friar Gregor Mendel used his studies of the reproductive lives of common pea plants to develop the foundations of modern genetics. Between Mendel's time and this very moment, scientists have worked ceaselessly to unlock our genes' secrets. Here is a primer on what we know to date.

The nucleus of every cell in your body (except red blood cells) contains forty-six chromosomes, twenty-three from your mother and twenty-three from your father. Each chromosome is made of bundles of deoxyribonucleic acid (DNA) and contains all the genetic information your body needs to develop in the womb and maintain itself after you've been born. Genes are specific sequences of DNA subunits that determine physical or biological characteristics, such as your height, eye color, and predisposition to certain diseases. The roughly twenty thousand genes influence health through the ways they express themselves, age, and mutate.

Mutations (permanent changes to a gene's DNA sequence) may be inherited from parents, occur during cell division, or be triggered by environmental factors. They are usually benign and occasionally even helpful. Charles Darwin's theory of natural selection, for example, is based on the idea that helpful mutations spark the evolution of species. Sometimes, however, good DNA goes bad; such mutations can lead to diseases, including cystic fibrosis, Tay-Sachs, and cancer.

The science of health and the science of genetics eventually found common ground, and today, most geneticists believe that our genes contain a blueprint of our health. Mutations, often passed down through generations, are responsible for many grave ailments. For example, in 1995, scientists discovered that a hereditary or "germ line" mutation was associated with high rates of breast cancer in American Jews. Another cancer-causing mutation occurs in as many as 1 percent of Americans, giving them a threefold to eightfold higher chance of getting breast, lung, stomach, skin, and pancreatic cancer.

Sometimes it's not what genes do, but what they *don't* do that affects people's health. In 1994, scientists working with mice isolated the OB gene, which sends hormonal signals to the brain telling us we've eaten enough. A mutation on the OB gene makes it difficult to gauge when we're full and is thought to be responsible for some types of obesity.

Losing weight is supposed to help prevent heart disease, but that may not be true if you're already genetically predisposed to it. In 2007, two separate studies found that a certain gene mutation can cause anywhere from a 30 to 64 percent increase in the likelihood of having heart disease. Both studies estimated that around 20 to 25 percent of Caucasians carry this mutation. Even if they maintain a healthy lifestyle, these individuals still have an elevated risk for heart attacks.

Such facts may make it seem as if our genes are ticking time bombs that can explode at any moment, striking us with cancer or some rare disease. However, a new branch of science called epigenetics holds that our genes operate in tandem with external conditions such as diet, stress, environment, and maternal nutrition. One way they do that is through a process known as methylation, which increases or decreases a gene's expression through exposure to certain nutrients.

Epidemiological studies have shown that over- and under-nourishment during a woman's pregnancy can cause health problems in her offspring. Perhaps the most famous of these studies was the Dutch Famine Study, in which scientists examined the effects of starvation during pregnancy on children conceived during the World War II Dutch famine known as "Hunger Winter." As adults, the women's offspring experienced high rates of heart disease, diabetes, and mental illness thought to be due to a lack of methylation in the genes they received from their undernourished mothers.

Too much methylation can be just as problematic as too little. A 2008 study showed that adults who had committed suicide after being abused or neglected as children had extra methylation in the DNA of cells of the hippocampus, one of the key areas of the brain associated with emotional function.

Daily stress also compromises the genes that control the immune system. A 1990 study indicated that stress dampened the ability of medical students' disease-fighting white blood cells to recognize viruses and bacteria. If stress is chronic, research shows, it can actually shorten the structures at the tips of the chromosomes, called telomeres, causing cells to age faster.

Telomeres protect genes against harm and organize them into correct position. Each time a cell divides, its telomeres shrink slightly. When they get too short, the cell ceases to function. This shrinkage likely underlies the haggard appearance of people who lead stressful lives—and the remarkable aging process seen in two-term American presidents.

The jury is still out on the immutability of our DNA. One scientific camp says we are slaves to it; the other, that our environment can modify it. One thing is certain: In order to stay healthy, we need to pay attention to what our genetic inheritance predicts and respond accordingly. If high blood pressure runs in your family, eat a low-fat, low-sodium diet; if breast cancer is common, women should have regular mammograms after age forty to catch malignant growths before they become life threatening.

These historical precedents need not doom us, however. Taking good care of your health may prevent whatever genetic possibilities seem to be in store from ever developing. You may not be able to control the genetic mutations you've received from your parents, but evidence increasingly shows that you *can* reduce the risks they pose.

Share in the Secret

If there's one secret you really can't share in, this may be it—unless you've found a way to go back in time and select parents with better genes. True, some religions that believe in multiple lives feel that in each incarnation you can choose your mother and father, but even then, it will be a lifetime before you receive another choice.

On the more scientific side, however, the newest avenues of research offer hope that we can alter our telomeres. In a recent interview with *The New York Times,* Dr. Elizabeth H. Blackburn, winner of the 2009 Nobel Prize in Medicine, called these structures "the protective caps at the ends of chromosomes," comparing them to shoelace tips: Much as laces fray and come apart when shoelace tips are lost or broken, truncated telomeres can damage our health. Because of the way they limit the lifespan of cells, shortened telomeres have been linked to age-related ailments.

So here's the good news: A recent study of thirty men with prostate cancer (conducted in part by Blackburn and her co-Nobel Prize–winning scientist, Carol Greider) showed that three months of eating a low-fat, plant-based diet, along with engaging in moderate exercise and stress management, increased the subjects' telomerase activity by almost 30 percent within a certain type of immune cell. The amped-up activity prevented the telomeres from deteriorating, which, according to the study, may help prevent these cancers from spreading.

In other words, this study, as well as many others, offers evidence that our genetic makeup is not necessarily fixed. Moreover, epigeneticists believe that our external environment can actually change it. Dr. Bruce Lipton, author of *The Biology of Belief* and a former medical school professor and research scientist, asserts that genes and DNA do not control our biology; rather, they are controlled by signals outside the cell. If this hypothesis turns out to be accurate, it's all the more reason to send your DNA the best messages possible by eating well, exercising, and trying some of the other secrets in this book.

SECRET

12

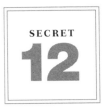

Herbal Remedies

LI CHING-YUEN

In May 1933, both *The New York Times* and *Time* magazine reported the death of a very old Chinese man named Li Ching-Yuen. Just exactly *how* old was a matter of debate: Li Ching-Yuen claimed to have been born in 1736, which would have made him 197 at the time of his death.

A few Chinese scholars, believing the man had forgotten his real birthday, went to work to figure out the truth. Not long afterward, Professor Wu Chung-Chien of Minkuo University produced a birth certificate proving that Li could not have been 197 as he claimed. He was actually 256 years old.

The only undisputed fact about Li's life is the date of his death. The rest of his story is a pastiche of legends, rumors, and tall tales cobbled together from shadowy sources. The legend goes something like this: Li was born in Chyi Jian Hsien in the mountainous Szechuan province of China in either 1677 or 1678; the birth certificate supposedly attests to that. Li spent his first seventy years hiking around China, gathering and selling medicinal herbs. Along the way, he also became a master of the martial art *qi gong* and began supplementing his diet with herbs, including ginseng, Asiatic pennywort, and Chinese wolfberries.

When he reached seventy-one, Li moved to Kai Hsien to work in the Chinese army as a tactical advisor and martial arts teacher, a position he held for roughly 170 years. In 1927, General Yang Sen invited Li to live with him so that he might study Li's secrets to extraordinarily graceful aging.

Yang's subsequent report, "A Factual Account of the 250-Year-Old Good-Luck Man," described Li as having very long fingernails and a ruddy complexion (long fingernails were a common trait among Chinese men of the era; being 250 years old was not).

Li returned home a year later to live with either his twenty-fourth or fourteenth wife, depending on who did the counting. It was there that *The New York Times* caught up with him, reporting that many of the old-timers in Li's neighborhood swore that Li had spent time with their grandfathers and that he had been a very old man even then.

When Li died, he left behind, besides 180 supposed descendents, a simple axiom for longevity: "Keep a quiet heart, sit like a tortoise, walk sprightly like a pigeon, and sleep like a dog." He also claimed it was the Chinese herbs that had kept him living—not only for more than a century, but also in the best of health.

The Facts on Herbs

Herbal remedies, long derided by the Western medical establishment, are an integral part of Chinese medicine. A growing body of research is proving that even if Li wasn't 256 years old when he died, he was right about the health-promoting powers of herbs.

The term *herbal remedies* refers to plants purported to have medicinal properties; these plants may well have been the first medicines ever used and studied by humans. Even today, approximately one quarter of all prescription drugs are derived from various plant-based sources, such as shrubs and herbs.

Although there are about a half million different plants growing on the earth today, only a fraction of them—approximately five thousand— have been studied for their medicinal benefits.

This paucity of research is largely because the wide availability of plants means they cannot be monetized as easily as invented prescription drugs. Still, the range of what we know plants may do is impressive, from alleviating high blood pressure to stimulating the nervous system, from destroying pathogenic microorganisms to boosting the immune system.

And they're remarkably easy to come by. Let's examine the facts behind a sample meal containing plants that heal as well as nourish.

Start with the beverage: green tea, a staple of Li's diet. Green tea, along with black, white, and oolong teas, is made from the leaves of the *Camellia sinensis* plant and has been used medicinally in China for at least four thousand years. When Western doctors finally got around to studying it, they found that the tea is packed with antioxidants called catechin polyphenols, in particular epigallocatechin gallate (EGCG).

The job of antioxidants is to destroy the body's free radicals, which damage cells, alter DNA, and contribute to chronic disease. In clinical studies, the polyphenols in green tea have been shown to boost metabolism and help burn fat, protect against liver disease, control blood sugar levels, lower bad cholesterol, and raise good cholesterol. The polyphenols also inhibit the growth of cancer cells in animals, and some studies point to similar benefits in humans.

Li is said to have drunk another herbal remedy, popularly known by its Sri Lankan name, gotu kola (*Centella asiatica*). Gotu kola, a cousin of parsley, is native to wetlands in many parts of Asia, South Africa, and the South Pacific. According to the American Cancer Society, studies have shown that it can improve poor circulation and help reduce the leg swelling brought on by varicose veins and poor circulation. When applied topically, chemicals in gotu kola called triterpenoids promote the healing of cuts and minor burns. Some evidence also suggests that gotu kola can slow the growth of tumors.

Still another beverage that might accompany our healthy herbal meal is ginseng tea. Few herbs are as controversial as ginseng—mostly because of the extensive claims its advocates put forward. But the benefits seem to be real: Many studies have shown that ginseng has antioxidant and liver protecting properties, as well as being an immune-system booster, although there is contradictory data regarding the liver.

Moving on to the soup course: Many Asian soups (notably Thai) are flavored with lemongrass, a time-honored remedy that is also a common ingredient in soaps, insect repellent, and candles. It is widely used not only for its citrus scent and flavor, but also because it is a potent antibacterial, containing geranial and neral, known antimicrobial agents. A recent study published in the *Internet Journal of Microbiology* showed that lemongrass oil can inhibit the growth of many types of harmful microbes.

To add some spice to the soup, throw in some cayenne pepper. Both whole and as a spice, this herb has been used to treat gastrointestinal disorders and promote heart health. There is some evidence to support cayenne's cardiovascular benefits and, oddly enough, a recent study showed that eating the potent red spice can benefit those suffering from heartburn. In addition, cayenne pepper is rich in vitamins A and C, the B vitamins, carotenoids, calcium, and potassium.

For the main dish, consider a stew flavored with ginger, a root that not only adds flavor but also helps soothe the stomach. Ginger's phenols (a class of chemical compounds) aid in digestion and relax the stomach muscles. According to the American Cancer Society, multiple studies have shown ginger's effectiveness in relieving stomach pain and nausea, especially if it is pregnancy related. It can also relieve chemotherapy-induced nausea, according to recent research by the National Cancer Institute.

Finishing off the meal, try a rhubarb compote spiced with cinnamon. Native to Asia, rhubarb has been used for thousands of years to treat stomach ills. The dark-red stalks are also filled with antioxidants that maintain healthy blood circulation, as well as vitamins C and K, which contribute to bone health.

Cinnamon, once said to be cultivated from the nests of phoenixes, has been proven to have natural antibacterial properties. Studies have shown that its oil can be an effective antibiotic against certain dangerous *Streptococcus* strains. And by combining cinnamon bark, lemon oil, and eucalyptus, you can create an ancient hand sanitizer called "thieves oil," so named because it was used by grave robbers in the Middle Ages to keep them infection-free after handling pungent corpses.

As noted earlier, despite thousands of years of anecdotal evidence and what we do know about the properties of certain plants, there is still a dearth of double-blind clinical trials demonstrating the efficacy of herbal and other plant remedies. And some of the tests that have been conducted produced results that were inconclusive at best—and at worst, showed the substances to be dangerous for human consumption.

Due to these untested or unproven health claims, in America herbs are marketed as "health supplements" rather than as drugs, meaning the regulations governing them are less strict. This distinction has created a very large market of relatively unknown goods, some of which can be harmful if taken improperly or without a full understanding of their potential interactions with other herbal supplements and/or prescription drugs. In Europe and Asia, however, herbal remedies are considered more mainstream, and are often sold at drugstores alongside prescription drugs. In many countries, such as England, herbalist schools are funded by the state government.

A 2008 study published in the *Journal of the American Medical Association (JAMA)* found that nearly 21 percent of 193 herbal supplements purchased online from sites purporting to sell Ayurvedic remedies contained dangerous substances including lead, mercury, and/or arsenic. In 2005, the American Association of Poison Control Centers received 5,334 reports of adverse reactions to dietary supplements, including vitamins, oils, and herbs.

HERBS AND FOOD

◆

Herbs mix well with food. They don't always mix well with medicines. According to a 2010 article in the *Journal of the American College of Cardiology*, certain varieties may interfere with common heart drugs, as well as other blood-related medicines. For instance, garlic and ginger may increase the risk of bleeding in patients who are taking blood thinners, and Saint-John's-Wort, typically taken to relieve depression, can raise both blood pressure and heart rate. However, the Council for Responsible Nutrition, an herbal product industry trade association, says the article represents a "biased, poorly written and contrived attack on herbal supplements." The bottom line: Although the data are still inconclusive, treat herbs as you would any other potent medicine or supplement, and use them responsibly.

Still, business is booming: According to the *Nutritional Business Journal*, in 2008, sales of herbal supplements in America were $25.2 billion, a gain of more than 6 percent over the previous year.

Share in the Secret

The secret to unlocking the power of herbs lies in ingesting sensible amounts of the right kinds. Returning to the elements from the herbal meal: When drinking green tea, the healthiest kind to enjoy is unflavored loose leaf, as opposed to bagged. Tea in bags has been more finely chopped, causing the leaves to lose freshness and nutrients faster. Regular tea contains twice as many catechins (antioxidants) as decaffeinated tea, three times more than flavored tea, and ten times more than bottled tea.

Ginseng is available in many different forms; the effectiveness of a ginseng product depends on the concentration and variety of ginsenosides (the active healthy compounds) within. As with other herbal remedies, there is no regulation as to the potency of the herb in the package you

THE PURPLE CONEFLOWER CRAZE

◆

If you've spent time outdoors in the United States anywhere east of the Continental Divide, the odds are good you've already brushed past some echinacea plants. Commonly called the purple coneflower, echinacea, found in the central and eastern United States, was long used as a cure-all by North American Plains Indians. Western doctors first adopted it as part of a late eighteenth-century movement known as eclectic medicine, which relied heavily on botanical cures, deriving many remedies from Native Americans. The eclectic doctors prescribed echinacea for everything from snakebites to anthrax poisoning.

Echinacea continued to be widely used well into the first quarter of the twentieth century until the 1928 discovery of penicillin helped diminish its popularity—as well as that of other herbal drugs. However, it has made a comeback over the last decade and is now widely used by herbalists, homeopaths, naturopaths, and others to help fight the common cold.

But does echinacea work? Scores of studies have proven inconclusive. The opposition cites a study by the University of Virginia, reported in 2005 in the *New England Journal of Medicine,* that concludes: "Extracts of *E. angustifolia* root, either alone or in combination, do not have clinically significant effects on infection with a rhinovirus or on the clinical illness that results from it." Proponents cite a 2007 metastudy assessing fourteen previous studies in the medical journal *The Lancet: Infectious Diseases,* which concluded that echinacea "decreased the odds of developing the common cold by 58 percent . . . and the duration of colds by one to four days."

Both of these studies have been harshly criticized by the opposing camps. One of the primary differences between the two was that that they were looking at different kinds of echinacea. The University of Virginia study was analyzing *E. angustifolia;* the other looked at many others, especially *E. purpurea.* Although *angustifolia* was used by the Native Americans, *purpurea* is now considered to be the species with the most health benefits. This is also the species that the German government recommends to fight off the common cold; its research on the plant has found that it also has antiviral, antibacterial, and anti-inflammatory properties.

buy, so talk to experts or search out reputable information on the Web. For the patient, buying the root itself might make the most sense. You can make a tea with it by brewing the root for an hour or so in a teapot. Other people chew on the ginseng root itself, although boiling it for ten minutes will make it more palatable.

Fresh lemongrass is available in most supermarkets, as is ginger. Whereas the latter can be employed widely in many different types of cooking, lemongrass is at its best chopped and used with other aromatic herbs such as chili, garlic, and cilantro. The outer leaves of the stalk are too tough to eat, so remove them to reveal the whitish purple center before cooking with it.

The active medicinal ingredient in cayenne pepper is capsaicin, present in all chile peppers. If you do not want to add the fiery red pepper to your food, try milder chile peppers to add spiciness without so much heat.

With rhubarb, as with any food that contains high quantities of fiber, special care must be taken not to eat too much, which can cause diarrhea. Also, due to its natural tartness, it is often cooked with a great deal of sugar, negating its natural health benefits. Instead of sugar, try stewing chunks of the stalk in fruit juice for a low-calorie treat.

Besides its usefulness in baking, cinnamon is also very effective in bringing out and deepening savory flavors. Instead of consuming it in the form of cinnamon buns and apple pie, add a pinch to soups or winter vegetables such as carrots and squash.

Innumerable other herbs can be used for both preparing food and protecting your health. Many come in pill form, but whether or not the pills are as effective as the actual herbs is in dispute.

Because the full medicinal powers of herbs, as well as their possible side effects, are not known, proceed with caution. You may want to consult a professional herbalist to select the plants that are most appropriate for you: Many websites can help you find an herbalist, such as those run by the American Herbalists Guild, the British Herbal Medicine Association, the European Herbal & Traditional Medicine Practitioners Association, or the National Herbalists Association of Australia.

Hydrogen Peroxide

BILL THOMPSON

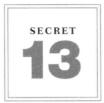

Want to sink a hole in one? Is your car looking dull? Sick of your unsightly stretch marks? Do you, or does anyone you know, own a Ginsu knife?

But wait! There's more! Home security devices, real estate opportunities, products to defeat body odor—if you've ever watched late-night television, the odds are good you know the work of sixty-three-year-old Bill Thompson. After a diverse career spanning a variety of jobs and locations, Bill currently owns and runs TV Inc., a Clearwater, Florida–based consulting firm whose mission is helping companies bring their products to market through infomercials; *products* can mean anything from a slicer/dicer to a candidate for the American presidency.

Bill has deep respect for the people with whom he agrees to work, but less for some of the other potential clients who come to him with ideas he calls insane. One man's scheme was a stock-rental company: If you couldn't afford to buy a stock, you could rent one for a period of time. Bill quickly reminded him of several people who were sent to prison for this practice.

Another man showed up with a "batteryless" ballpoint pen. "Have you ever seen anything like it?" he asked. "Here's a Bic," Bill replied. The man was incensed. "I'm going to sue them," he fumed.

Another rejected concept was essentially a portable toilet seat, invented by a woman for people who feel uncomfortable touching the seats in public restrooms. Still, some may find Bill's own health routine pretty unusual—dunking his head in hydrogen peroxide.

He first learned about peroxide from researcher and hydrogen peroxide expert Kenneth Seaton, MD. Among other things, Seaton's studies found that when the beneficial bacteria in your system encounter harmful bacteria, they excrete a little bit of hydrogen peroxide to destroy them. Thus, the thinking goes, hydrogen peroxide is a natural germ killer.

So each morning Bill pours a coffee cup's worth of hydrogen peroxide into a sink filled with lukewarm water, shuts his eyes, puts his head in the sink, and blows bubbles through his nose to get the mixture circulating. "Standing naked, my face in the water, I hope no one is behind me, because it's not a pretty sight," he says.

Bill credits the routine for his perfect health; he hasn't had even a cold in more than two decades. At his last physical, his doctor told him he had the EKG of a twenty-year-old. Bill takes it one step further: "When you take your face out of the water, you feel like you're eighteen years old."

The Facts on Hydrogen Peroxide

Making rocket fuel; removing earwax; whitening teeth; bleaching hair; cleaning countertops, clothes, vegetables, and fruits—the applications of hydrogen peroxide are myriad, although its most prominent use is in the American paper industry to bleach and process pulp.

THREE UNUSUAL HEALTH SECRETS

Unlike hydrogen peroxide, a few health claims for some unusual or unlikely remedies *are* undergoing study here and abroad. Here are three of the strangest:

MAGGOT DEBRIDEMENT THERAPY (MDT)

Centuries ago, field personnel noticed that wounded soldiers whose injuries were maggot-infested healed faster than those whose wounds were not. Doctors came to realize that the maggots (fly larvae) consume dead tissue while leaving healthy tissue alone. They also secrete matter that can restrain and even kill bacteria.

More than fifty scientific papers have been published that describe the medical use of maggots, six

thousand maggot-therapy patients have been included in case histories, and about four hundred patients have participated in clinical studies of the creepy crawlers. The results were impressive enough that in 2004 MDT was declared an FDA-approved medical device.

FIRE CUPPING

In this technique, a bell-shaped, approximately four-fluid-ounce cup is placed on a patient's back after the cup's interior has been heated with fire, creating a vacuum as glass connects with skin. From eight to twelve such cups are arranged in two parallel columns, then removed after about twenty minutes. According to the American Cancer Society, this

Soon after the compound was first isolated in 1818 by a French chemist, uses for hydrogen peroxide proliferated. As the above list suggests, most were nonmedical until, in 1920, the British medical magazine *The Lancet* reported the promising results of a treatment for patients with influenza involving hydrogen peroxide infusions.

In the 1940s, Father Richard Willhelm, founder of Educational Concern for Hydrogen Peroxide, a nonprofit organization dedicated to educating the public on the safe use and therapeutic benefits of the substance, reported that the compound could be used as a treatment for everything from skin disease to polio. Today, its practice is "recommended mainly for treating bronchial congestion, arthritis, and pain. It is also promoted to ease depression and reduce swelling." However, the Society states that "available scientific evidence does not support claims that cupping has any health benefits."

URINE THERAPY

Sometimes called the world's oldest medicine, urine therapy, or uropathy, refers to the use of one's own urine to enhance health, usually by drinking or massaging it into your skin. Millions of people swear by its efficacy. Performer Madonna once explained on *Late Night with David Letterman* that she cured her incessant athlete's foot by urinating on her own feet in the shower. Actress Sarah Miles has drunk her own urine for three decades,

claiming it cures allergies. It is said that Indian leader Mohandas Gandhi believed in uropathy as well.

Practitioners of urine therapy, called uropaths, claim that "oral autotherapy" drinking one's own urine—inoculates humans against many forms of cancer. This assertion is based on the logic that cancer cell antigens are expelled through urine, and by introducing them back into the immune system, the body is encouraged to create preemptive antibodies.

There's little scientific evidence for uropathy, but it is being studied. One of the roadblocks, however, is the difficulty in setting up solid blind experiments. It's hard to hide the fact that test subjects are drinking urine, as opposed to a placebo that smells and tastes like it, and few people want to drink someone else's.

advocates claim it can treat even more problems: clogged arteries, cancer, ear infections.

Less controversial is how hydrogen peroxide works to heal surface wounds such as insect bites and canker sores: It breaks down when exposed to air, releasing free radicals in the form of oxygen atoms. These free radicals then oxidize and kill any nearby bacteria, disinfecting the skin. And according to Bill Thompson, unbroken, peroxide-protected skin can fight off all invaders.

Who knows? Little research has been done on hydrogen peroxide, in part because it cannot be patented and therefore can't be a lucrative source of revenue to anyone. Like herbs and hydrogen peroxide, many health secrets with thousands or even millions of supporters have scant formal scientific proof behind them. These remedies range from Bach flower drops to aromatherapy, from homeopathic potions to evening primrose oil. Such treatments based on commonly available substances may or may not prove efficacious for a given individual, but as far as broader populations are concerned, we may never know whether they really work unless large-scale tests are conducted.

That may never happen, but what research exists is being aided and monitored by a U.S. government agency. Due to the level of interest in alternatives to conventional Western medicine—40 percent of Americans say they use them—in 1991 the U.S. National Institutes of Health (NIH) created a special division, the Office of Alternative Medicine. In 1998 the office was reestablished as the National Center for Complementary and Alternative Medicine (NCCAM).

NCCAM is the federal government's lead agency for scientific research on medical and health care systems, practices, and products not generally considered part of the mainstream. The NCCAM finances investigations looking at how various alternatives affect healing. Current projects include studying the effects of tai chi on osteoporosis in women and those of acupuncture on chronic pain.

Until NCCAM research produces more results, perhaps the best way to judge treatments for which there is little to no medical proof is on a case-by-case basis. On one hand, lack of scientific proof doesn't mean the remedy is necessarily ineffective. On the other, there is plenty of snake oil around on which to throw away money, and some alleged cures have caused serious harm—for example, Radithor, an early twentieth-century cure-all consisting of distilled water and a tiny amount of radioactive radium. Radithor was advertised as "perpetual sunshine," but led to perpetual darkness for some users, such as the steel baron Eben McBurney Byers, who died only a few months after his first swig.

Share in the Secret

If you want to try a hydrogen peroxide regime, Bill's formula is simple: Pour a cup of hydrogen peroxide into a basin of lukewarm water and, eyes closed, duck your head in. Blow bubbles through your nose. Dry off afterward. Don't worry about your hair: The hydrogen peroxide is too diluted to bleach it.

Remember, however, that hydrogen peroxide is H_2O_2, not H_2O. Its vapors can be potentially dangerous; concentrated doses can be very corrosive, and even low doses can bleach clothes if spattered on them. Most important, it is dangerous if swallowed: As it decomposes in the stomach it releases large quantities of gas, potentially causing internal bleeding.

Just to be extra safe, keep the twenty-four-hour phone number of the National Poison Control Center (1-800-222-1222) posted prominently in your home.

Lifting Weights

SASHA LODI

A quick glance at Sasha Lodi tells you little. He has a powerful frame despite his below-average height; his thick hair is solid black, but his face is weathered and creased. He could be from a Latin or Mediterranean culture, and his age might be anywhere between forty and sixty.

He's actually a seventy-three-year-old Tibetan weightlifter.

Sasha's parents left his native city of Lhasa in 1947 during political unrest and moved to Karachi, Pakistan. His father was a doctor of homeopathy; his mother reared Sasha and his seven brothers and sisters. The family relocated to Europe, living in England, France, and Italy before finally settling in Ontario, Canada, where Sasha attended college, earning a degree in organic chemistry, "which I've never used."

Instead, he entered the fitness business, ending up in New York City, where he first worked for a health spa and eventually started his own high-end line of clothing called, naturally, Sasha. Tiring of fashion, in 1988 he returned to the gym as a trainer at the Excelsior Club on Manhattan's Upper East Side; twenty-two years later, he's still there. In the meantime, he got married and had two children.

His health has been excellent throughout his life, a fact he attributes to strength training. Sasha started lifting when he was sixteen to help him gain strength for playing cricket and soccer, and has kept it up for fifty-seven years. There was even a time when he was a competitive bodybuilder, winning the titles of Mr. Junior Pakistan and Mr. Montreal.

Despite the workouts, Sasha did have one period in his life when he wasn't healthy. After "forty years of living like a monk," in the 1980s he—like many others—fell into the New York disco scene and a routine of dancing, drugs, and debauchery. The birth of his son in 1988 snapped him out of that.

These days, he's at the gym seven days a week, training approximately eight people a day, and himself five of those days. To help his body recover from the effort, he exercises different body parts on different days, completing a full-body cycle once a week.

Weightlifting is good for health, he says, because it increases the metabolism more than any other activity and also increases muscle mass. "This is the prime difference between being old and young. If you have the same muscle mass when eighty as when you're thirty, few changes will take place in your body. Any form of exercise is good, but cardio by itself just does the heart. It does not address the muscles," he explains.

Diet is important, too. Sasha practices a "90/10 ratio": 90 percent good food, 10 percent whatever he feels like eating. However, he never uses sugar or white flour, nor does he drink coffee, preferring tea for its theanine—an amino acid that purportedly helps lift the spirits. On those rare occasions when he feels he might be coming down with something, he eats garlic and drinks organic apple cider vinegar, a mixture he finds cleansing. And, like many strength trainers, he takes "every vitamin known to man," as well as a host of other supplements, including saw palmetto, pygeum, CoQ10, alpha-lipoic acid, DHEA,

DUMBBELLS, SOUP, AND BALLS

◆

The most important factor in any weight training regimen is overload—that is, lifting more weight than your muscles are prepared to lift. The perfect amount of weight lets you complete the desired number of repetitions but no more.

You don't need iron for overload: Anything that offers resistance against your muscles can work. This allows for creativity. Soup cans and water bottles are substitutes for dumbbells, or, for the stronger, gallon milk jugs filled with water or sand. If you don't have any such objects handy, overload can also be achieved by exploiting the effect of gravity on your body. For instance, exercises like push-ups, pull-ups, crunches, and leg lifts can be considered forms of weight training without the external weight. After all, look at gymnasts, whose exercise routines involve strength training using only their bodies. But if you really want to feel the burn, try combining bodyweight exercises with free weights, such as push-ups with a bag full of books on your back, or crunches with a medicine ball cradled against your chest.

fish oil, glucosamine and chondroitin, and turmeric. He also downs a daily health drink composed of protein powder, flaxseed oil, wheat germ oil, pumpkin seed oil, glutamine, ester-C powder, brewer's yeast, and creatine monohydrate in a liquid base created by boiling fresh ginger, fresh turmeric root, cinnamon, and green tea in a gallon of water, plus some pineapple juice for taste.

The Facts on Lifting Weights

The phrase *pumping iron* may be new, but strength training isn't. Chinese texts dating back five thousand years describe weightlifting tests that trainee soldiers were required to pass to join the army, and ancient Egyptian tombs depict people using bags filled with sand and stone for lifting and throwing. Competitive weightlifting was a major part of the early Olympic Games; among the games' most famous athletes was the wrestler Milo of Croton, said to have trained for the games by carrying the same calf on his back every day for four years, even as the calf grew into a much heavier cow.

Not long after Milo, Hippocrates uttered one of the most enduring axioms of strength training: "That which is used develops, and that which is not used wastes away."

In modern times, we've traded animals for iron as the weight of choice. In the early twentieth century, the invention of the adjustable barbell made weightlifting more practical and efficient, and as the equipment evolved, so did the science behind strength training. Athletics coaches noticed the correlation between strength training and enhanced sport performance; it soon became part of physical education programs.

> "THE BEST ACTIVITIES *for your health are pumping and humping."*
>
> ARNOLD SCHWARZENEGGER, GOVERNOR OF CALIFORNIA, FORMER CHAMPION BODYBUILDER

A critical advancement in strength training came in the 1970s with the introduction of Nautilus equipment, machines that brought resistance training into the mainstream. Unlike free-weight training, resistance training uses tension instead of raw mass to build muscle, reducing the need for an array of weights. Think arm-wrestling or opening a stubborn pickle jar.

Despite the continuing development of equipment and medical knowledge about its benefits, strength training remains a niche form of exercise. As of 2006, only 20 percent of American adults were doing strength training at least twice a week—a slight increase in that number over the previous decade has been chalked up to women picking up weights in greater numbers. Those who do it swear by it, but most people prefer cardiovascular exercise.

Unlike running (see Secret 20, page 149), strength training is a form of *anaerobic* exercise—exercise that works the muscles at a rate faster than that at which your body can supply them with oxygen. Anaerobic exercise tends to be short and intense; a typical activity usually lasts less than a minute, at which point the body's lactate and hydrogen ions start hampering the muscles' ability to keep exercising.

Advocates like Sasha claim a long list of benefits for anaerobic exercise, most of which are preventive. According to the Department of Kinesiology and Health at Georgia State University, these benefits include reducing the risk of premature death, heart disease, high blood pressure, high cholesterol, colon and breast cancer, depression, and diabetes, as well as reducing body weight and body fat. Moreover, it can help build and maintain healthy muscles, bones, and joints. Increasingly, strength training is thought to be critical for seniors, helping to develop lean muscle mass and bone strength and maintain a high metabolic rate. In other words, strength training can lower a person's biological age. As Sasha says, research confirms that the major commonality among people who live long lives is their ability to retain muscle mass. This ability suggests a capacity to grow and repair lean muscle, which requires a high metabolic rate—something strength training promotes. In addition, strength training releases natural human growth hormone, which is critical in rejuvenating the body, providing energy, and fortifying the immune system. By strengthening bones, it also can be highly beneficial to menopausal women, who often fall victim to osteoporosis.

While strength training offers a variety of advantages, it's important to be prudent. All anaerobic exercise is intense and often requires pushing the body to new limits. This kind of workout routine may be risky for certain people—and not just because of the possible muscle strains, leg cramps, and badly performed exercises that lead to pulled tendons and ligaments—all of which happen to those who aren't paying attention. A recent study in the *JAMA* has suggested a link between weight lifting and serious cardiac problems, pointing to five healthy young people who suffered "aortic dissection," splitting of the aorta walls, which creates an extremely harsh pain and is lethal without immediate attention. Aortic dissection is thought to be related to elevated blood pressure. In a healthy adult, systolic blood pressure is typically around 120 mm Hg (millimeters of mercury); during intense

SITTING DUCKS

Some people prefer anaerobic exercise; others, aerobic; but perhaps the most important move is to stand up. In a 2010 article published in the *British Journal of Sports Medicine*, Elin Ekblom-Bak of the Swedish School of Sport and Health Sciences asserts that sitting for prolonged periods of time may be highly detrimental to your health, even if you regularly exercise during those times you're not seated. It seems the more you sit, the more likely you are to be in poor health.

According to a 2009 report on seventeen thousand Canadians studied for more than ten years, the more time people spent seated, the higher their death risk, whether or not they exercised regularly. Furthermore, a recent Australian study revealed that for every extra hour women spent sitting, their risk of metabolic syndrome—a precursor of diabetes and heart disease—rose

by 25 percent, regardless of their exercise regime.

Ekblom-Bak writes that, after four hours of sitting, the body starts to send harmful signals that cause genes regulating the amount of glucose and fat in the body to start shutting down. Similarly, a 2010 Australian study of almost nine thousand adults found that each hour of television viewing was accompanied by an 18 percent increase in heart disease and an 11 percent increase in overall mortality. (According to the lead researcher, it is highly likely that the act of sitting still for four or more hours is more injurious to health than the television programming.)

The antidote? Don't sit in one place for more than forty-five minutes. Get up. Walk around. Sit down again. Get up again. Drink some water. Walk up and down a flight of stairs. Sit again. Get up. Go the bathroom. Sit. Repeat.

weight training, pressure can rise to 300. Dr. John Elefteriades, chief of cardiothoracic surgery at Yale–New Haven Hospital, who headed the *JAMA* study on aortic dissection, states, "Our research and findings indicate that there is a very real health danger for people who lift exceedingly heavy weight due to the increased stress that it places on the aorta."

SEX AND HEALTH

◆

Another form of exercise for many (and for some, their only form) is sexual intercourse. Eastern cultures have long considered sex essential for healthy living. Chinese Taoists envisioned sex as the merger of two people's energies. The Hindu philosopher Mallanaga Vatsyayana wrote the famous *Kama Sutra* to instruct people in more fulfilling, healthy sexual practices.

In America, however, sex has been historically viewed as shameful. Puritan immigrants to the New World carried with them the biblically influenced belief that the human body was inherently impure, and that following its desires leads to sin, although the sex act itself was not frowned upon as long as it occurred within the confines of marriage for reproductive purposes.

Despite this cultural hangover, most twenty-first-century Americans are more liberal in their attitude toward sexuality, an acceptance that may be boosted further by recent reports indicating that sex not only creates life but also helps prolong it. Studies have linked sex to a variety of health benefits, including stress relief, strengthened immune function, increased cardiovascular health, decreased risk of prostate cancer, better self-esteem, reduced chronic pain, and deeper sleep.

Part of this benefit derives from the way sex works the heart (exercise-wise); for example, a 2002 report of a study of British men found that the

Share in the Secret

Danger lurks in an overambitious weight-lifting program, in focusing too much on challenging a single body part, choosing ineffective exercises, and performing exercises incorrectly.

Always follow sound principles when strength training. Here are a few basics:

- *Select appropriate and efficient exercises.* For example, doing one squat takes the same amount of time as one leg extension, but does more for your body.

physical effort involved in performing sexual intercourse can provide protection from fatal coronary events, and many other studies corroborate these findings. Benefits come not only from the exercise involved but also from the end result. Generally speaking, the more orgasms we experience, the better. In a recent study linking sex to improved prostate health in men, it was found that it didn't matter how the men climaxed, just that they did so often. Some studies have even suggested that sex may be a biological fountain of youth. Each time a person reaches orgasm, levels of the hormone dehydroepiandrosterone (DHEA) in his or her body rise. DHEA is associated with maintaining healthy skin and tissue as well as improving cognition.

Although a wealth of data now links sex and good health, it's not clear which is responsible for which. "We know that healthier people have more sexual activity," says Jennifer Bass, who is the director of communications at the Kinsey Institute for Research in Sex, Gender and Reproduction in Bloomington, Indiana. "What we don't know is: Does good health make you more willing to have sex, or does the sex have a positive impact on health?"

It may be that the health benefits of sex actually derive from the stable, loving relationships in which it occurs, and not from one-night stands. Sex researchers still have a lot to prove, but as yet no one has collected any data proving that safe and responsible sex is bad for you. On the other hand, bad sex probably isn't much good for anyone.

- *Monitor the frequency of your workouts.* The idea behind strength training is to stretch the muscles to the point at which they need to be rebuilt and allowed to grow. Thus, construct strength training routines around short, intense workouts a day or two apart to allow recuperation. (Some studies suggest that muscle can continue to grow as much as a week after a workout.)

- *Select the right type of set.* A set is a series of repetitions of a given strength exercise at a certain weight. Some trainers recommend single, high-intensity sets that lead to muscle exhaustion; others advocate multiple sets at a slightly lower intensity. Both set styles lead to similar strength gains, but research shows that single-set workouts can confer that benefit in less time.

• Above all, do not start strength training without some kind of expert guidance.

If you decide to start a weight-training program, consider joining a gym and asking a trainer for help in doing the exercises properly. If you can afford it, hire one, at least to learn the basics. Or read the fairly technical but fact-filled book *Strength Training Anatomy*, by Frederick Delavier, which explains everything you need to know and provides graphics showing how to do it.

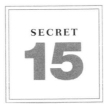

SECRET
15

Napping

SARNOFF MEDNICK

I n 1997, Sarnoff Mednick was standing at a podium at a conference
of the American Psychiatric Association, giving a lecture on children
at high risk for schizophrenia. As he was speaking, papers propped
in front of him, he suddenly fell asleep.

Normally Sarnoff takes a nap or two each day, but he hadn't had
the time before this particular talk. So habituated to snoozing was
he that his system apparently went ahead and fell asleep midspeech.
Luckily, as he drifted off, Sarnoff's body slouched over the podium, and
as he tilted forward, he woke up, found his place in his speech, and
continued as if nothing had happened. A friend who knew that Sarnoff
took regular naps had noticed the pause, but no one else seemed to—at
least, no one admitted it.

Sarnoff, who has a PhD from Northwestern University and a medical
degree from the University of Copenhagen, is currently professor emeritus

SMART NAPS

◆

According to new research from the University of California at Berkeley, naps not only improve your health, they make you smarter. In an experiment with thirty-nine young adults, one group napped for ninety minutes; the other didn't. The former then scored far better on learning tests. Such results corroborate data from the same research team about students who stay up all night to cram for exams—it's not a good idea: The lost sleep apparently decreases the ability to learn new facts by nearly 40 percent, due to a shutdown of brain regions during sleep deprivation.

of psychology and director of the Social Science Research Institute at the University of Southern California. He is an expert on schizophrenia, a mental disorder he has been studying most of his life. He's also an expert on naps, which he has been taking for most of his life. The habit started in graduate school, when he would go to the library to study but become drowsy and fall asleep at the table. An afternoon nap soon became an intentional routine, although no longer indulged in at a library table.

Sarnoff claims napping is the primary reason why he never comes down with colds and flus, and that's why he continues to do it. These days, however, his age gives him an excuse to doze that he never had before: Now he can just say, "I'm eighty-two years old. I need to take a nap"—no questions asked. And although he prefers a comfortable couch, he can fall asleep on the floor. Actually, "I can fall asleep anywhere now."

Normally his naps last about a half hour, but sometimes longer. Regardless of length, Sarnoff says, they always refresh him; some days, he takes two. It makes him feel better, and he finds that after waking, he gets quickly back to speed on a project, performing even better than before the nap.

Sarnoff did have one serious health incident. One day in 1983, he felt chest constriction. Recognizing the danger signs of heart disease, he went to his physician and was soon undergoing a bypass operation. He recalls that the condition arose because, despite his doctor's warnings, he was also regularly consuming large quantities of fat and cholesterol. Today he watches his diet, exercises daily—twenty minutes on a treadmill plus twenty minutes of weight training—and continues to nap.

Besides helping him maintain good health, Sarnoff's napping has had another unintentional but powerful effect: inspiring a career. When his daughter, Sara, was studying for a PhD in psychology at Harvard, she worked closely with Robert Stickgold, an expert on nocturnal sleep. Needing a niche of her own, Sara was inspired by her father's lifelong dedication to the afternoon nap and decided to focus on that area; eventually she became one of the field's leading experts. "If it weren't for my dad," she says, "I wouldn't have thought of something as obscure as nap research as a specialty."

The Facts on Napping

Of all the reasons to be asleep at noon, the best might be to avoid the wrath of Poludnica (Lady Midday). According to Eastern European lore, if she catches you out in the fields on a hot summer day, she'll give you heatstroke, drive you crazy, or lop off your head with a scythe.

The myth of Poludnica is a little extreme, but it represents a primordial human disdain for being awake at midday. Our affinity for lying low when the sun is at its highest originated before the advent of recorded history. When humans still lived in isolated, seminomadic groups, they were *polyphasic* sleepers—sleeping in multiple short periods over a twenty-four-hour stretch—as a matter of necessity. It was too dangerous for the entire group to sleep for long periods of time without someone keeping watch for predators. Although we developed an attachment to night sleeping when we began living in small societies, we didn't abandon the midday kip. Instead, we became *biphasic* sleepers—sleeping for one long period during the night and one short period during the middle of the day. The ancients even established the

SLEEPING WITH THE ENEMY (OF SLEEP)

According to research by sleep specialist Neil Stanley, MD, of the University of Surrey (U.K.), sharing a bed with a partner is not necessarily a healthy idea for either party— especially when the partner is male.

Between restless limbs, snoring, and disagreements over what time to set the alarm, one study found that couples suffered an average of 50 percent more sleep disturbances if they shared a bed than if they slept solo.

Dr. Stanley pointed out that the tradition of sharing a marital bed is relatively new, dating from the Industrial Revolution, when population growth meant more people with less furniture. In ancient Rome, for example, the marital bed was used only for sex, not sleeping.

And according to sociologist Robert Meadows, PhD, also at the University of Surrey, "People actually feel that they sleep better when they are with a partner, but the

noon nap as an institution that the Romans called *hora sexta,* the "sixth hour" past dawn, that is, twelve o'clock.

The tradition of napping began to decline in thirteenth-century Europe due (historians believe) to the invention of the mechanical clock, which changed people's perception of time by dividing it into discrete units. Gradually, workers started getting paid by the hour rather than by the job—meaning there was no time for naps. Many centuries later, the demands of the Industrial Revolution exacerbated this trend, codifying the concept of an uninterrupted workday in most parts of the world (except certain societies in warmer climates, such as Spain and India).

Despite the current stigmatization of napping as a slothful habit, history is awash with accomplished nappers. Leonardo da Vinci was a polyphasic sleeper, preferring a series of short naps every few hours to prolonged nightly rest. Napoléon Bonaparte often couldn't get a good night's sleep due to the pressures of war, so he dozed on his horse.

evidence suggests otherwise." When Meadows studied how well couples slept sharing a bed versus sleeping separately, his results showed that when couples share, and one of them moves in his or her sleep, there is a 50 percent chance that his or her partner will be disturbed.

Scientists at the University of Vienna have even found that men who share a bed may temporarily reduce their brain power, as it is likely to disturb their sleep, impairing not only their mental ability but also increasing their stress-hormone levels the next day. According to the same

study, women who share a bed fare better because they seem more able to cope with broken sleep patterns. This ability is due in part to the necessity to adapt to sex-specific life events, such as nursing babies and menopause, which create sleep disruptions but to which women seem biologically predisposed to acclimate. Of course, this study didn't look into the effects that male snoring has on their bedmates.

Scientists conclude that if you're successfully sleeping with someone, fine; if not, there is no shame, and much to gain, in sleeping apart.

Thomas Edison was also an inveterate napper, and an unapologetic Winston Churchill once said, "Nature had not intended mankind to work from eight in the morning until midnight without the refreshment of blessed oblivion which, even if it only lasts twenty minutes, is sufficient to renew all the vital forces."

Whether you nap or not, you are spending about one third of your life asleep, although scientists don't really know why. Our need for sleep is "the biggest open question in biology," says Dr. Allan Rechtschaffen, sleep expert and professor emeritus at the University of Chicago. What *is* clear is that all of us have what's called a basal sleep need: We require a certain amount of sleep to be healthy, but that amount varies according to age and individual. And if we do not meet our basal sleep needs, we accumulate a sleep debt that can adversely affect our health.

Sleep deprivation has the same biological effect as stress: Overtired bodies ratchet up production of the hormone cortisol, which lends us energy but restricts production of human growth hormone, which limits the body's ability to repair itself. And just like stress, sleep loss has a degenerative affect on our health.

Also like stress, lack of sleep is connected with compromised immune function. A 2008 Stanford University study revealed that the immune system of fruit flies fought invading bacteria hardest at night, a finding consistent with the long-standing hypothesis that our bodies spend dormant hours regenerating and fighting off disease through the production of immune cells called monocytes. Without enough sleep, says a study from the University of California, San Diego, the number and effectiveness of immune cells decreases.

> "THERE IS ONLY ONE THING *people like that is good for them: a good night's sleep."*
> ~EDGAR WATSON HOWE, AMERICAN NOVELIST AND EDITOR

Sleep shields us from more than just the common cold, as shown by a recent University of Chicago report revealing that lack of sleep can promote calcium buildup in heart arteries. This buildup can, in turn, lead to heart attack and stroke. The study found that as little as an hour less sleep than we really need can increase coronary calcium levels by 16 percent.

Although many people associate lack of sleep with weight loss, the opposite is true. There is a well-proven correlation between shorter sleep times and increased body mass index, but until recently researchers didn't know why. Then, in 2004, a Stanford study demonstrated that light sleepers had reduced levels of the hormone leptin and elevated levels of the hormone ghrelin. This chemical imbalance increased the appetite of those with short sleep cycles, contributing to their obesity.

Convinced? But not convinced that you have time to nap? This is a misconception, according to Sara Mednick, who is currently a research scientist at the Salk Institute in La Jolla, California. In her book, *Take a Nap! Change Your Life,* she explains how people can fit naps into their schedule with a little planning and a better understanding of their sleep patterns.

To begin with, you have to understand that sleep is divided into five stages:

- Stage one

- Stage two

- Short-wave sleep (SWS), comprising stages three and four

- Rapid eye movement (REM), stage five

A given sleep stage can be achieved only by passing through the previous stages, and each has its own regenerative properties. Nappers should be concerned primarily with reaching stage two, SWS, and REM sleep. Sara Mednick calls stage two the "stock" of the sleep soup, because "not only does it provide the medium in which all the other stages 'float,' but it's also pretty nutritious all by itself." This stage is responsible for increasing alertness and, because it occurs relatively early in the sleep cycle (after two to five minutes of stage-one sleep), is easy to access.

However, if deeper rest is necessary, an SWS nap is key. Mednick says that the critical physical benefits of sleep take place during this phase. Since it follows stage two, any nap longer than twenty minutes will give you an extra boost of SWS.

REM is the final stage of sleep and, like the other stages, helps enhance memory and perceptual skills. The amount of time you're likely to spend in REM, as well as in SWS, varies depending on the time of day you close your eyes. An entire sleep cycle takes roughly an hour and a half and will always include different periods of both stages.

The optimal time to nap is between one and three in the afternoon. Not only is this a period when our bodies are most in need of rest (assuming we rise at dawn), but also a ninety-minute nap during these hours offers the optimal proportions of stage-two, SWS, and REM sleep.

Despite the plethora of health benefits linked to napping, at least one study casts some doubt on its efficacy: In 2009 a study presented at

Diabetes UK's annual professional conference in Glasgow reported that those who nap were 26 percent *more* likely to get type 2 diabetes than those who didn't. The study suggests that napping may disrupt nighttime sleep (important for warding off this disease) and is correlated with reduced physical activity. Still, there's accumulating evidence that an afternoon nap may be exactly what Mednick thinks it is—a quick and refreshing step toward good health, as well as an excellent means of avoiding the wrath of Poludnica.

Share in the Secret

Here are a few simple tips to help you nap wherever you may be:

- Don't forget to go to the bathroom beforehand. It's hard to sleep when you have to go.

- Find a safe, quiet place out of the light. This might mean closing the door to your office and shutting the blinds, or perhaps just putting in earplugs and placing a shade over your eyes.

- Remove anything that will prevent you from relaxing, including textbooks, tools, company reports, computers, and above all, telephones—especially your cell phone.

- Make sure you're warm, but not so warm that you will oversleep your allotted wake-up time. (At night, you might want to consider a cooler temperature.)

- Find a comfortable posture that supports your neck and limbs. If lying down is impossible, try to elevate your legs. However, it's estimated to take about 50 percent longer to fall asleep sitting upright.

For some, clearing the mind is also essential. Try repeating a mantra to eliminate bothersome thoughts, or picture yourself far away from your home or office in your favorite quiet place—a forest glen, a remote beach.

If you have some control over your napping environment, you might consider adding a lavender-scented candle or basket of potpourri, since aromatherapists say the smell of lavender helps bring on sleep.

Here's a final, counterintuitive tip: Consider drinking a cup of coffee or a caffeinated beverage right before your nap. Because it will take about twenty minutes for the caffeine to travel through your digestive system, you can fit in a short snooze before it takes effect. Japanese research found that subjects who imbibed caffeine just before a nap were more alert when they awoke than those who didn't, and their ensuing work productivity was high.

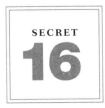
pH Balance

THOMAS APPELL

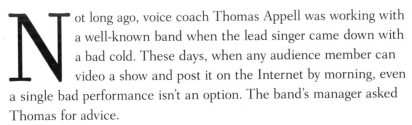

Not long ago, voice coach Thomas Appell was working with a well-known band when the lead singer came down with a bad cold. These days, when any audience member can video a show and post it on the Internet by morning, even a single bad performance isn't an option. The band's manager asked Thomas for advice.

Thomas's response—his standard riff on pH balance—may not have been what the band was expecting, but they listened to him explain what to eat and what not to eat. They then devoured a salad wrap (see page 124) that he prepared for them in his kitchen, and then watched (and listened) as the singer recovered his voice. A day later, Thomas got another call; the band had already forgotten how to make the wrap. "Weird as it sounds," their manager told him, "this salad is going to help us sell records."

Until 2002, Thomas himself had a bad history of colds and flu, getting nailed two or three times a year. The illness hindered his work as a vocal coach: It's hard to teach others when you sound like a frog.

Thomas has been involved with music for most of his life. When he was ten, his parents, devout Christians who adopted him at birth, enrolled him in trumpet lessons. The next year he joined a vocal group called The Choralaires and appeared on the television show *Church in the Home.* Soon thereafter he began guitar lessons and formed a band, Love's Perfection; their first gig was at a Taco Bell. By 1982, he'd been in two popular groups; when one of the band members left (eventually joining the band Mötley Crüe), Thomas began his voice training career.

Twenty years later, a terrible sore throat made him realize he had to find a way to restore his health. His doctors had told him to take antibiotics or other medications, but he resisted: "I didn't want to address the symptom. I wanted my system to be healthy." So he, like me, decided to track down the secrets of people who never got sick.

One of those people was Mike, a voice student who'd grown up on a farm in Ireland. The reason Mike and his entire family were so healthy, he claimed, was the food and water they consumed. They never ate sugar or meat, and the water they used to irrigate their garden came from a spring flowing through a limestone shelf loaded with calcium.

Thomas started eating as Mike did—no sugar, no meat, more vegetables—and felt good enough to continue his research. After conducting a two-year study, he decided he'd found the underlying reason Mike's protocol worked. His system was being alkalized (as opposed to being acidified) by his diet—he was eating four alkaline nutrients for every acidic one.

"Viruses, cancer, and most diseases don't survive in an alkalized environment," Thomas says, but "they thrive on anything acidic. The key to good health is to make sure that you are eating [predominantly] alkaline food to keep your body balanced."

Thomas routinely checks his urine pH after a meal to see the food's effect on this balance. "Your health is entirely dependent on your acid/base levels," he maintains. "If you don't know your pH balance, you don't know your health."

The Facts on pH Balance

Remember sitting in high school chemistry class, watching beakers heating over a flame, staring at the periodic table on the wall, and dipping little strips of paper into solutions to test something called pH?

The term pH means "potential of hydrogen," or the concentration of hydrogen ions in a particular solution or medium. When there is an excess of hydrogen ions, the solution's pH is acid. Too few hydrogen ions means the solution is alkaline.

The pH is measured on a scale from 0 to 14, with 0 completely acidic, 14 completely alkaline, and 7 neutral. Water is more or less neutral, though its precise pH depends on the source. Acid rain is, as you might guess, very acidic.

As Thomas maintains, the human body has an optimal pH level. On the whole, the body works best when the blood is slightly basic, or alkaline, around 7.4. It must remain around this level to function properly.

To understand the claims of those who think pH balance in diet is important, consider the theories of Antoine Béchamp, one of the heroes of alternative medicine. Béchamp was a contemporary of Louis Pasteur, whose experiments helped prove the germ theory of disease, which posits that most diseases are caused by microscopic invaders, specifically bacteria and viruses. Béchamp disagreed, arguing that germs are the by-products of disease, rather than the cause.

According to Béchamp, the body is healthy when its internal systems are pH balanced. It is subject to disease only under certain conditions, during which the otherwise benign microscopic organisms inhabiting the body in periods of good health are transformed into germs. Instead of a germ theory of disease, think of a disease theory of germs.

SOME COMMON ACIDIFYING AND ALKALIZING FOODS

◆

ACIDIFYING

Corn oil, sunflower oil, barley, corn, oats, rice, wheat, butter, cheese, milk, cashews, peanuts, walnuts, bananas, blueberries, grapes, oranges, peaches, plums, pineapple, strawberries, beef, chicken, fish, turkey, alcoholic beverages, coffee, sugar

ALKALIZING

Olive oil (cold-pressed), asparagus, broccoli, cabbage, carrots, cauliflower, celery, garlic, lettuce, onions, peas, peppers, spinach, avocados, lemons, limes, tomatoes, lima beans, lentils, soybeans, almonds

Today's pH advocates believe that the healthy balance Béchamp advocated can be obtained by monitoring food intake. When pH levels fall below 7.36, the body suffers from a condition called acidosis, and when the level rises past about 7.42, it enters what is called alkalosis. Both conditions can be harmful depending on their severity, but acidosis is more common and has a greater variety of causes.

Two major types of acidosis exist: respiratory and metabolic. Respiratory acidosis occurs when the lungs cannot remove sufficient carbon dioxide from the body. Metabolic acidosis may occur when the kidneys can't process acids fast enough. Acidosis may be caused by kidney failure, diabetes, and even severe malnutrition. In mild cases, symptoms include fatigue, rapid breathing, gastrointestinal problems, and confusion. In severe cases, the disease is deadly.

If you remain skeptical, think about acid rain. Caused by the chemical pollutants sulfur dioxide and nitrogen oxide reacting with the water vapor in the air to form acids, it is harsh and harmful to plants, animals, and even buildings. Or imagine cooking an egg in a cup of hydrochloric acid—it would simply disintegrate. Highly acidic substances are harmful to life—and they are all around us, affecting us all the time.

Many pH experts believe that acidosis is an epidemic of the modern world—and not just from our environment. According to naturopath Christopher Vasey, author of *The Acid-Alkaline Diet for Optimum Health,* the shift away from a plant-based, low-protein diet toward a diet high in meats and sugars has had a negative impact on public health.

Eaten regularly, advocates say alkalizing foods can reduce the risk of bodily acidification. Most vegetables are alkalizing, especially leafy greens, but raw and cooked green beans, asparagus, carrots, and collards are safe bets as well. And some fruits are alkalizing, including cucumbers, coconuts, and avocados. (Oddly, more obviously acidic foods have a less cut-and-dried impact on bodily pH. Yogurt, some citrus fruit, and tomatoes can be perfectly healthy choices in a pH-balanced diet.) As for beverages, water is the best choice, followed by vegetable and wheatgrass juices.

Several recent bestselling books, including those of microbiologist Robert O. Young and medical anthropologist Susan E. Brown, PhD, examine the relationship between disease and metabolic acidosis. In her book *Better Bones, Better Body,* Brown claims that the acidifying diet common to contemporary Western society promotes metabolic acidosis. One of the diet's most severe effects is a loss of bone mineral, leading to osteoporosis and other common bone-related afflictions.

Not everyone agrees that pH balance is something people should monitor—or even think about. Dr. Mark Liponis, medical director of the Canyon Ranch health resort, says, "I find this idea kind of funny. It's like saying, 'The key to good health is keeping your temperature at 98.6, or keeping your blood sugar between 70 and 100 or your potassium at 4.0.' Our bodies do this automatically; we regulate pH closely. I think it would be hard to change or control even if you wanted to. For example, if we ate something very acidic, our breathing rate would increase to get rid of the extra acid as CO_2 and our kidneys would spill acid. That's a normal, automatic, unconscious process."

Still, Liponis and other critics add that the changes people make to improve their pH balance—eating more fruits and vegetables, less processed food, less sugar, and fewer refined carbohydrates—are very healthy in and of themselves, so even if you aren't convinced that pH balance is the key to health, its recipes make sense.

Share in the Secret

The first step to attaining optimal pH levels is knowing what yours are; you'll need to test your urine for that. Visit a drugstore or go online and buy litmus paper—narrow, absorbent strips used to measure pH, like the ones from high school. Follow the directions, including holding it in the flow of your urine for a couple of seconds. The strip will change color; compare that color to those on the pH chart included with the litmus paper.

Urine pH should hover around 7—neutral, like water. Don't worry if it shows up acidic or alkaline now and then, but if one extreme or the other becomes a trend, something may be wrong.

According to Robert O. Young's *The pH Miracle: Balance Your Diet, Reclaim Your Health* (written with Shelley Redford Young), the keys to perfect pH are drinking at least four liters of pure water daily; eating highly alkaline foods—such as vegetables and certain fruits—while avoiding meat, chicken, fish, sugar, and grains; and taking supplements, such as certain baking salts.

Most often, however, a shift toward pH balance comes from a change in overall lifestyle, not just diet. For example, appropriate levels of exercise can increase energy and improve metabolism; physically active people have an easier time oxidizing acids. Stress is also a major cause of acidification, resulting in both bad moods and poor health. Says Dr. Young's website, the human body produces more acid when it's under stress, and also has a more difficult time counteracting it. Stress makes the heart work harder as well, straining the circulatory and pulmonary systems. Therefore, it's a good idea to avoid stress whenever possible (see Secret 22, page 166) and to find outlets to relieve the stress you're already undergoing.

TOM'S SALAD WRAP THAT SAVED THE BAND

◆

Large handful of washed raw
   spinach leaves

Small handful of mixed greens

Small handful of sesame seeds

10 blueberries

½ cup buckwheat groats

¼ bell pepper, chopped

1 avocado, sliced

½ mango, sliced

¼ sour green apple, sliced

5 strawberries, sliced

3 inches of cucumber, sliced

1 kiwi, sliced

1 Roma tomato, sliced

A few shakes each of Litehouse brand
   freeze-dried garlic and basil

Mix ingredients together in bowl. Add dressing to taste—Tom prefers extra virgin olive oil. To make a wrap, take a ten-inch Fat Flush tortilla (Tom's favorite brand, because it contains sprouted grains), roll it into the shape of an ice cream cone, and stuff in as much salad as possible.

YIELD: *Because the salad is so big, Tom eats it twice—a portion in the morning as a wrap, and the leftovers later in the day with a fork.*

Plant-Based Diet

RIP ESSELSTYN

Firefighters are known for their intensity and courage while fighting a fire—and also for the games they play and bets they make while dealing with their downtime. At Engine 2 Company in Austin, Texas, the firefighters like to see who can climb the pole fastest hand over hand without using their feet, or who can hoist the 180-pound dummy over a shoulder, carry it up the back stairs, through the dormitory, and down the front stairs in the shortest amount of time.

Back in 2006, when forty-five-year-old former firefighter Rip Esselstyn and his friends JR and Josh were chatting about their health, they quickly made a bet on whose cholesterol was lowest. When they found out that JR's was dangerously high at 344, Rip sprang into action, helping his colleague by guiding him onto a plant-based diet. Not long after the change, JR's cholesterol level fell below 200.

For many years, Rip, a former University of Texas All-American swimmer, was one of the world's top triathletes: first place, the 2001 Police and Fire World Games; first place, the Capital of Texas triathlon (eight times); and a top-three finisher in the Escape from Alcatraz triathlon.

> "I'D LOVE TO TELL *all those critics how well I feel today because of my diet. But they're all dead.*"
>
> ~ROBERT CUMMINGS, AMERICAN ACTOR AND HEALTH FOOD ADVOCATE, WHO SAID, "NEVER EAT ANYTHING WHITE"

When he joined the Austin Fire Department in 1997, Rip quickly learned that most of the calls a firefighter answers aren't fire-related—somewhere between 70 and 80 percent of them result from some kind of medical emergency, from car accidents to fainting episodes, from truculent drunks to diabetics in insulin shock. Rip and his team spent more time resuscitating people and performing CPR than they did spraying water through hoses.

This means that firefighters are constantly being exposed to one disease after another, from people who are sick with the flu or a fever to those who cough and vomit on them, or, occasionally, die in their arms. But Rip never missed a day of work. His secret: a diet of grains, vegetables, fruits, and legumes. "It's a diet that's light on calories and heavy on nutrients, which is the opposite of how most Americans eat: heavy on calories and light on nutrients. I fortify my immune system by loading up on all the vitamins, minerals, and phytochemicals found exclusively in these plant-based foods. Without them, I'd be sick as a dog."

Rip is such a persuasive advertisement for his notions that he convinced his entire shift at the fire station to eat just plants, making them the only group of plant-eating firefighters in the country—even if the next shift, composed of meat-eaters, did once place beef bouillon cubes in all the showerheads.

I know about Rip because I was part of his first study on lowering cholesterol through diet: The group also included several firefighters and a wide range of people from housewives to athletes to white-collar professionals. After following Rip's diet for six weeks, every one of us who completed the study saw our total cholesterol and LDL (or bad cholesterol) levels fall. My own cholesterol level dropped from 240 to 170, my LDL from 139 to below 100.

I then co-wrote Rip's book, *The Engine 2 Diet*, which caught the attention of John Mackey, CEO of Whole Foods, who consequently hired Rip away from the Austin Fire Department to start a line of Engine 2 Diet foods for his customers who need help becoming plant-based cooks.

The Facts on a Plant-Based Diet

Sometimes it's not what you eat but what you don't eat. Plant-eaters like Rip do not consume any food that comes from a member of the animal kingdom. That means no meat, no fish, no milk, no eggs, no cheese, and no butter. For hardcore vegans, this also means no honey, as honey comes from bees. For truly hardcore vegans, it refers to clothes as well they refuse to wear leather, wool, and fur, as these items are derived from animal skins

The term *vegan* was coined in 1944 by Britons Elsie Shrigley and Donald Watson, who used the first three and last two letters of the word vegetarian because they saw veganism as the beginning and end of vegetarianism, and they disliked the notion that vegetarians ate dairy and other animal-based foods. Vegans, they decided, should not use any animal products, in any way, such as in clothing or shelter.

Today the majority of vegans are still driven by animal-rights concerns, but an increasing number are health-conscious, believing that consumption of animal fats and proteins causes a wide variety of illnesses, including heart disease, colon and lung cancer, osteoporosis, diabetes, kidney disease, and hypertension.

A 2006 Harris Poll on Americans' food choices showed that approximately 1.4 percent of respondents kept vegan diets, which amounts to more than two million U.S. vegans.

WERE OUR PREDECESSORS VEGAN?

◆

Although the term *vegan* was coined in 1944, it seems likely that humans didn't eat many animal-derived foods until the advent of controlled fire some 800,000 years ago. Before that, archeological evidence suggests that humans might not have had the correct dental apparatus necessary to chew tough, raw meat.

Eight hundred thousand years may seem like a long time, but since *Sahelanthropus tchadensis*, the oldest known hominid, lived 7 million years ago, meat entered the human diet relatively late in the evolutionary process.

Furthermore, humankind's ancestors, primates, are also largely vegan. A seminal Harvard University paper on contemporary primate diets references animal consumption only briefly in a category called "miscellaneous," and claims that the 5 percent of nonvegetable foods in primate diets includes termites and other insects (rather than meat)— insects often eaten accidentally while the primate is consuming plant food.

Is veganism the natural human state? The truth is, no one really knows. Should it be? The man who probably understood animal behavior better than anyone else, Charles Darwin, once said, "The normal food of man is vegetable."

For years, little research was done on the effect of a plant-based diet on health. Then, in the mid-1980s, several studies showed that such diets had promising benefits, especially when it came to preventing heart disease, stroke, Alzheimer's disease, and cancer.

One of the first such studies was carried out by Rip's father, Dr. Caldwell Esselstyn, a surgeon at Ohio's Cleveland Clinic and, in 2005, the first recipient of the Benjamin Spock Award for Compassion in Medicine. His twenty-year study, begun in 1986, showed that eating a low-fat, plant-based diet could arrest, and even reverse, heart disease. At the same time, Dean Ornish, MD, was conducting his Lifestyle Heart Trial Study at the University of California at San Francisco; his results were published in 1991 in the medical journal *The Lancet*. Ornish's patients, placed on a low-fat, plant-based diet, saw a reverse in or an end to their preexisting arterial blockages, as well as a reduction in or elimination of their angina.

Some of the best data on plant-based diets come from Dr. T. Colin Campbell, Cornell professor and project director of the China-Oxford-Cornell Diet and Health Project, whose bestselling book, *The China Study,* chronicles the results of a thirty-year investigation of nutrition and health that

examined more than 6,500 people in sixty-five different Chinese villages. His results showed that the Chinese, who ate a predominantly whole-food, plant-based diet, were far less likely to suffer any kind of coronary disease than were Americans. And the results of the Framingham Study, the largest equivalent review of diet and heart disease among Americans, were comparable to those of the China Study.

Numerous other inquiries indicate a link between cancer and animal products, especially saturated animal fat, animal protein, and insulin-like growth factor 1 (IGF-1), a powerful growth-promoting hormone. Saturated fat suppresses the immune system and contains excessive calories, both of which spur growth of all cells—even cancer cells. According to *The China Study*'s Dr. Campbell, the animal protein in dairy foods (even fat-free products) contributes to an acidic environment in which cancer cells and tumors thrive.

A June 1999 article in the journal *Alternative Medicine Reviews* reported that prostate cancer was more strongly correlated with the consumption of nonfat dairy products than with any other food product. In other words, it's not about the fat, it's about the dairy. And an eight-year study conducted in conjunction with the American Association for Retired Persons showed that people who ate meat frequently had a higher risk of several types of cancer—including lung, colorectal, esophageal, liver, and pancreatic cancer—than those who didn't.

Despite the positive news, veganism doesn't necessarily connote good health. In fact, vegans can be in terrible shape, because simply eating vegan isn't enough. Unless you are an intelligent eater and have access to a variety of fruits, vegetables, and legumes, and can also supplement your diet with the appropriate vitamins and minerals, you're not doing your body any favors.

For instance, there was a time when vegans could pick up the vitamin B_{12} they needed in the dirt attached to foods. Nowadays, with foods scrubbed antiseptically, that's not possible (see the hygiene hypothesis, page 50). Absence of vitamin B_{12} can cause anemia and neurodegenerative diseases, so vegans must eat foods fortified with B_{12}, or take a supplement of at least 500 micrograms daily.

> "A HUMAN can be healthy without killing animals for food. Therefore if he eats meat he participates in taking animal life merely for the sake of his appetite."
> ~LEO TOLSTOY, RUSSIAN NOVELIST

Similarly, vegans must be sure their diet includes enough calcium, which they can get from fortified soy milk and greens such as Swiss chard or kale; broccoli and almonds are also good sources. Between 500 and 1,000 milligrams a day should probably be enough, but everyone has different needs. Plant-based eaters should consider having their vitamin B_{12} and calcium levels tested.

Vitamin D, too, must be supplemented, either via exposure to the sun for about twenty minutes a day (this number varies widely, depending on your skin pigment and your location), from foods fortified with Vitamin D, and/or from supplements. (Vitamin D levels in the United States are low for nearly everyone, vegan or carnivore.) A supplement should contain at least 400 IUs (see page 183 for more on vitamin D).

Share in the Secret

Those who would like to try a plant-based diet for a month can visit Rip Esselstyn's *Engine 2 Diet* website. There you can find hundreds of vegan recipes as well as a monthly meal plan.

If you want to start right now, it's easy: Simply cut out any food that comes from something that had a face or a mother. In other words, no cheeseburgers, fried clams, or omelets. But because this diet is highly nutritious and high in fiber, most people can consume all the vegetables, legumes, fruits, and whole grains they want without gaining weight.

But remember, you must be careful that your meals include all the vitamins and nutrients necessary to stay healthy.

For starters, here is a recipe that Rip and the firefighters love.

SWEET POTATO–VEGETABLE LASAGNA

Preheat oven to 400°F.

1 large onion, chopped

1 small head garlic, all cloves chopped or pressed

8 ounces mushrooms, sliced

1 head broccoli, chopped, without stems

2 large carrots, chopped

2 red bell peppers, seeded and chopped

1 can corn (15 ounces), rinsed and drained

1 package firm tofu (16 ounces)

½ teaspoon cayenne pepper

1 teaspoon oregano, preferably fresh

1 teaspoon basil, preferably fresh

1 teaspoon rosemary, preferably fresh

2 boxes (8 ounces each) whole grain lasagna noodles, uncooked

2 jars (25 ounces each) pasta sauce

1 pound frozen spinach, thawed and drained

2 sweet potatoes, cooked and mashed

6 Roma tomatoes, sliced thin

1 cup raw cashews, ground

Sauté the onions and garlic on high heat for 3 minutes in a wok or nonstick pan. Add the mushrooms and cook until the onions are limp and the mushrooms release their liquid. Remove them to a large bowl using a slotted spoon. Reserve the mushroom liquid in the pan. Sauté the broccoli and carrots for 5 minutes, and add them to the mushroom bowl. Sauté the peppers and corn until just beginning to soften, and add them to the vegetable bowl. Drain the tofu by wrapping it in paper towels. Break it up directly in the towels and combine it with the vegetable mixture. Add the cayenne and herbs to the vegetable bowl and stir to combine.

PYTHAGOREANS

◆

While veganism is still fairly rare, somewhere between 5 and 9 percent of Americans are vegetarians, meaning that like vegans, they don't eat meat or fish, but they do consume dairy products and eggs. The term vegetarian is only about 160 years old; it was coined in 1847 in Britain for the newly organized British Vegetarian Society. Until then, vegetarians were called Pythagoreans, after history's first prominent vegetarian, the Greek philosopher Pythagoras (c. 570 to c. 495 B.C.), who founded a philosophy based on mathematics.

Pythagoras said, "As long as man continues to be the ruthless destroyer of lower living beings, he will never know health or peace. For as long as men massacre animals, they will kill each other."

Pythagoras also said, "In a right triangle, the square of the hypotenuse is equal to the sum of the squares of the other two sides."

TO ASSEMBLE: Cover the bottom of a 9 × 13-inch casserole with a layer of sauce. Add a layer of noodles. Cover the noodles with sauce. This way the noodles cook in the oven rather than being boiled first, saving time and energy. Spread the vegetable mixture over the sauced noodles. Cover with another layer of noodles and another dressing of sauce. Add the spinach to the second layer of sauced noodles. Cover the spinach with the mashed sweet potatoes. Add another layer of sauce, the final layer of noodles, and a last topping of sauce. Cover the lasagna with the thinly sliced Roma tomatoes, then cover the dish with foil and bake in the oven for 45 minutes. Remove the foil, sprinkle the top with cashews, and return the lasagna to the oven for 15 minutes. Remove it from the oven and let it sit for 15 minutes before serving.

YIELD: *Serves 10 to 12*

Positive Attitude

GAIL EVANS

For many years, Gail Evans, then the executive vice president of CNN, flew all around the world on a regular basis. Once, when she traveled to Malta for the Bush/Gorbachev summit, her plane landed during a hurricane. The meeting itself took place on a ship at sea, the rain was pouring, the temperature was dropping, and everyone was soaking wet. When Gail came back to her hotel room, she had a chill and felt terrible. Nevertheless, she told herself, "You have five more days left at this event. You are not going to become sick."

She didn't. In fact, at sixty-eight, Gail can't recall taking a sick day from school or work. It's possible, she says, that she might actually have been sick at some point over the years. She didn't pay attention. "It's about attitude. I'm confident I'll never get sick, but if I do feel bad, I know I can conquer it immediately. Many people get a runny nose or a cough and think they're ill. I don't. I cough a little, I sneeze a little, but it doesn't stop me."

Gail, who no longer works for CNN but still lives in Atlanta, calls her medical health philosophy "benign neglect." Yet she says, "I'm not an idiot. If I found a lump on my body, I'd go to a doctor. If I were to break a leg, I'd get it fixed. But most people carry their health concerns too far. The moment something goes wrong, they run to the doctor's office and, given the litigious nature of our society, doctors feel they have to err on the side of doing more, not less, for their patients. So they find something wrong and announce the patient is sick."

Gail believes that the body is self-regulating and that although you'll have your ups and downs, you're more likely to *be* well if you *think* you're well. Gail's attitude began to form during the 1960s, when she and her family lived in Moscow. Her son Jason was two weeks old when they arrived. She soon became pregnant with her next son, Jeffrey. Only one American doctor was around at the time; his previous job had been on an aircraft carrier, and he knew nothing about women's health, much less obstetrics. The Russian doctors, Gail says, were not helpful. So when one of the American women fell ill, the others would pitch in and help out. They read every book they could and found that most people could survive in this manner unless a genuine medical crisis occurred.

"It's not that I ignore my health. If I hear an intelligent tip, I pay attention. If I walk into a room where everyone is hacking and coughing, I'm careful where I stand and whom I talk to. Still, I believe I can say to my body: You are *not* getting sick."

Gail does go in for a regular checkup. Her physician once told Gail that if she had to depend on patients like her, she'd go broke.

The Facts on a Positive Attitude

In the 1950s, a man referred to as "Mr. Wright" in medical literature was dying from cancer of the lymph nodes. Bedridden, with orange-size tumors spotting his body, he was barely able to breathe, and his doctors told him he had no hope of recovery. However, Mr. Wright had heard about a new medication called Krebiozen and pleaded with his doctors to give it a try. Although they doubted its efficacy, the doctors consented. Buoyed by the belief that his health had been repaired, within three days, Mr. Wright was wandering around the hospital, joking with the nurses, while his tumors shrank to half their previous size. Ten days later, he was discharged.

However, Mr. Wright soon read media reports questioning Krebiozen's usefulness. His attitude changed. He lost faith in the drug, he became despondent, and soon he suffered a relapse. So his doctors conspired to trick him back into health. They told him to ignore the press because they were going to give him a newer version, and a better dose, of Krebiozen.

There was no such thing. The doctors merely injected the man with nothing more than distilled water.

But believing once again that he could be cured, Mr. Wright's health improved dramatically, and he went home again. Unfortunately, after reading a report that ultimately debunked Krebiozen, he died within a day.

Another story: In 1994 Dr. Bruce Moseley of Baylor College of Medicine asked ten patients scheduled for operations to relieve pain in their arthritic knees to participate in an experiment. All ten would go through what seemed to be a complete operation, but only two would actually undergo the standard knee surgery; three would have part of it; five would have no surgery at all. But all would be treated so that they would believe they had received the full surgery.

None of the patients knew who had received the surgery, but after the procedures were performed, all ten reported much less knee pain. Simply thinking they had received the surgery proved as effective as actually having had it.

Mr. Wright's and Dr. Moseley's stories are among the best known in the annals of mind-over-body medicine, but they are only two among thousands.

Mind-body medicine claims that thoughts and emotions have the power to exert a positive (or negative) influence on physical health. This positive attitude can derive from any number of sources—a doctor's support, a placebo (an inert sugar pill), positive thinking, self-suggestion, and so on.

Belief in the mind-body connection is as old as Western medicine itself: As far back as the fifth century B.C., Hippocrates said, "The natural healing force within each one of us is the greatest force in getting well." Since then, the relationship between health and mind has been studied more than any other aspect of health. Many thousands of books have been written on the subject, along with scores of magazine and newspaper articles; Google the subject and 125,000,000 references pop up. The number of cases of people who feel cured of illness simply by believing they are well grows every day.

But does attitude truly affect health? No one can say for sure, because science has not yet found a definitive way to prove that attitude works. Certainly many people will testify that their attitude keeps them healthy, but many others are convinced that their attitude has had no effect whatsoever on their health. For every two studies showing the power of attitude, there's another one debunking it.

In *The Cure Within*, Anne Harrington's encyclopedic study of mind-body medicine, the author introduces readers to many centuries of experimentation and research into the subject. This research, however, turns up more questions than answers. Why do placebos work so well—sometimes better than the drug for which they've been substituted? Why do some people seem to become healthier by thinking positive thoughts more easily than others? Why does the power of suggestion seem so potent, but so impossible to prove?

For many years, science simply wasn't willing to tackle these questions. But sentiment has changed, due in part to a popular book. In the 1970s, editor Norman Cousins wrote the hugely successful *Anatomy of an Illness as Perceived by the Patient,* in which he told of curing his own life-threatening illness, diagnosed as severe ankylosing spondylitis. Cousins restored his health, largely by rejecting negative emotions, reading humorous books, and watching Marx Brothers movies and the old television show *Candid Camera*.

Soon after, Cousins was invited to join the medical faculty at UCLA, where he helped create the field of psychoneuroimmunology—the study of the relationship between the body and the mind. The concept was now firmly planted in the culture.

Another reason for the change is that other research has shown that substances naturally occurring in the body can cause alterations in mood as well as sensations of pain and pleasure. The chemicals, called endorphins, produce what's commonly known as a runner's high. In other words, processes are at work that are quantifiable and therefore can be scientifically studied.

Moreover, research on biofeedback has shown that people can control their own brain waves and change their cardiovascular and respiratory functioning using just their minds. And, studies in consciousness have revealed that some people can relieve their own headaches and lower their own blood pressure solely through willpower.

Over the last decade, attitude and belief have been proven to affect the course of many chronic illnesses, as well as day-to-day health. Studies at university research centers, at institutions like Yale and Rutgers, have shown that a person's attitude toward his or her health is possibly the best predictor of physical well-being. Published reports from 2009 showed that various mind-body techniques were able to successfully treat conditions such as fibromyalgia, cancer, and Alzheimer's; other studies have shown a connection between attitude and the successful relief of back and other kinds of pain, sleep disorders, inflammatory bowel disease, and celiac disease, among other ailments.

According to the National Kidney Foundation, positive attitude is considered an important factor in whether one's body will accept an organ transplant. And according to the National Institute of Arthritis and Musculoskeletal and Skin diseases (NIAMS), "perhaps the best thing you can do for your health is to keep a positive attitude" when treating osteoarthritis.

However, there have been challenges to some of the most prominent studies purporting to show a strong correlation between mind and body. Perhaps the most prominent of these involves the work of Stanford psychiatrist David Spiegel, whose 1989 *Lancet* article described the groundbreaking finding that support groups helped women suffering from cancer to live longer. Twelve years later, a new test was unable to replicate these findings, leading some to doubt the original results. Other mind-body studies have been challenged on different grounds, including accuracy of data and problems with methodology.

Furthermore, some medical personnel have not welcomed the positive-attitude approach toward health. They point out that if people are told that their attitude controls their health, but they then fall ill, it implies they have a bad attitude or are somehow mentally defective compared to those who don't get sick.

Attitude, after all, is not quantifiable, nor is it always controllable— today, at least. In the future, machines that can help us better manage our attitudes may hold the secret to human health.

Share in the Secret

Telling someone to "have a better attitude" is a little like telling yourself to be a better person. Easy to say. Hard to do.

What if you're someone who can't enhance your frame of mind despite your best efforts? Plenty of help is available. The proverbial power of positive thinking is one of the most popular themes in publishing. Some of the innumerable books on the topic include Norman Vincent Peale's 1952 blockbuster, *The Power of Positive Thinking,* and the recent runaway bestseller by Rhonda Byrne, *The Secret.* Most of the books in this genre are more popular with readers than they are with medical professionals.

If you're not a reader, you can try technology. Biofeedback machines can help you learn to consciously influence your body's responses and, in turn, your health. According to *Alternative Medicine:*

The Definitive Guide, so can several mind-body integration techniques, such as guided imagery, breath work, energy psychology, eye movement desensitization and eye reprocessing, meditation, and neurolinguistic programming.

Judith Orloff, MD, a practicing psychiatrist as well as assistant clinical professor of psychiatry at UCLA, is the author of the bestselling books *Positive Energy* and *Emotional Freedom.* She has spent much of her life trying to improve other people's attitudes. Here are her tips to improve yours:

1. Understand that beliefs set the tone for health and healing. Positive attitudes accentuate wellness; negative attitudes impair it. Our beliefs trigger biochemical responses. No organ system is apart from our thoughts. Beliefs set a tone for certain health realities to occur.

2. Try to focus on what's good in the Now rather than catastrophizing about what danger lurks in the Later. Negative fear-based thoughts increase the stress hormones in your body and stop the blissful flow of endorphins, our brain's natural pain-reducing neurochemicals.

3. Take a few minutes to meditate each day on a positive image: a waterfall, a sunset, the night sky, a child's face. This calms your physiological system and allows you to take a minibreak from the stressors of the day.

4. Practice positive self-talk. This form of affirmation will neutralize the tendency to focus on what is negative. For instance, if you're tired, tell yourself, "Honey, it's OK to take a rest," instead of beating yourself up for not moving nonstop. When you know you've done your best in a situation or are in the process of healing from an illness, say, "You've done a great job"—even if it's not perfect. This emphasis on what you've done well instead of what you've done wrong will help keep your body calm and healthy.

5. Be grateful for what is working in your life rather than obsessing on what has gone wrong. Always focus on the love you have and know the enormous value of this love.

6. Practice anonymous acts of service whenever you are feeling unhappy or in a bad mood. Reaching out to help others in a small way, such as helping someone across the street or being emotionally supportive of a friend, serves to open your heart and generate positive energy, so you feel better—and so does someone else.

Having a positive attitude is something that you practice over time. The more you get in the habit of doing it, the more successful you will be.

Probiotics

TONY JAPOUR

Infectious diseases have figured prominently in Tony Japour's life. First, they're the reason both his parents are deaf. His maternal grandmother contracted German measles (rubella) when she was in the second trimester of pregnancy, which resulted, as is common, in deafness in her unborn child. In his father's case, it was an earache in infancy that led to bacterial meningitis and his eventual deafness.

Second, one of Tony's closest friends died of AIDS, caused by the HIV retrovirus.

Finally, as a student at Northwestern University Medical School, Tony was most intrigued by the infectious-disease component of whatever he was studying. For example, while studying gastroenterology, he became interested in the viral pathogens that cause hepatitis; while studying cardiology, he was fascinated by the infections that cause myocarditis.

After receiving his MD, Tony took a residency at a community hospital affiliated with Harvard, stayed there for a fellowship studying infectious diseases, and chose AIDS research as his specialty. He eventually joined Harvard's faculty as a molecular virologist. Then, in 1996, he left to work at Abbott Laboratories in its AIDS drug development group, helping to develop Kaletra, a highly successful drug that changed the paradigm of AIDS treatment toward the use of protease inhibitors.

When not occupied by infectiousness, Tony has had other careers. While hoping to be appointed to head the FDA by President George W. Bush (it never happened), he set up a contemporary art gallery in Miami. A few years later, he became a politician, running for a seat in the Florida House of Representatives. Given his accomplishments (and his movie-star looks), in 2003 *People* magazine named him (along with Ashton Kutcher and Keanu Reeves) one of the country's twenty-five most eligible bachelors; Tony was the first to ask the magazine to mention that he was gay.

Although generally healthy, Tony used to come down with a nasty cold every year. For the past six years, however, he hasn't been sick at all, and he credits his routine morning concoction.

Once a day, in a teacup, he mixes pasteurized raw egg whites with a container of DanActive (usually the vanilla flavor). Tony credits his good health not to the product itself but to the active ingredient within, the bacterium *Lactobacillus casei* Immunitas. These bacteria are what's known as probiotics, or a type of microorganism beneficial to its host.

Tony's Lebanese grandmother always made yogurt from scratch and told him it was good for his health. It just took him about four decades to act on her advice.

The Facts on Probiotics

For half of the twentieth century, the word *antibiotic* was one of the most powerful in medicine. Coined in 1942, the term describes any substance produced by a microorganism that can stop the growth of or destroy other, harmful microorganisms.

The action of antibiotics was first described almost seventy years earlier by Louis Pasteur, who noticed that *Bacillus* could inhibit the growth of the harmful *Bacillus anthracis.* From his discoveries came the family of the most powerful and most frequently prescribed class of drugs of the last century, from penicillin to tetracycline.

When scientists figured out the mechanism by which certain substances could destroy harmful bacteria, euphoria followed. People assumed that all disease could be eradicated by this method.

It didn't happen. But because antibiotics have been enormously helpful in many areas of medical treatment, the notion of something called a *probiotic* can still surprise. We've come to think of bacteria as a bad thing, and we want to kill them all. But if we did, our bodies would be in a lot of trouble (see the hygiene hypothesis, page 50).

A healthy human's gastrointestinal tract is rife with billions of friendly bacteria vital to our health and well-being. As mentioned, there are between ten and twenty times more bacteria than cells in our body. Rather than causing disease, they prevent it, fighting viral infection and other ailments. The term *probiotics* was coined in 2001 by the Food and Agriculture Organization of the United Nations, which defines them as "live microbes which when administered in adequate amounts confer a health benefit on the host." The concept behind using probiotics is simple: helping our population of friendly bacteria do their job.

The person first credited with attempting to identify and explain the health benefits of bacteria-based supplements was the 1908 Nobel Prize–winning Russian scientist Ilya Mechnikov. Theorizing that the aging process—the gradual inability of our body's cells to make healthy replacements—is caused by the ravages of toxic bacteria in the gut, Mechnikov focused on finding ways to minimize their numbers. Eventually concluding that lactic acid, found in sour milk, helped suppress the growth of pathogenic (or disease-causing) bacteria, he put his theory into practice by drinking a glass of sour milk each day. It turns out sour milk *does* have beneficial properties. The bacteria in it, *Lactobacillus acidophilus*, produces vitamin K, lactase (which is essential to the digestion of lactose), and several antimicrobial agents.

Over the last decade, numerous studies have demonstrated the power of probiotics. For example, research conducted at the Jean Mayer U.S. Department of Agriculture Human Nutrition Research Center on Aging at Tufts University recently concluded that yogurt consumption can have a beneficial impact on many gastrointestinal conditions, including constipation, diarrhea, colon cancer, and inflammatory bowel disease. It can also help promote the body's natural defenses against infections.

Other studies have shown that probiotics boost the immune system, support urogenital health, lower blood pressure, decrease cholesterol, reduce symptoms of inflammatory bowel disease, and improve the body's ability to absorb minerals.

In November 2005, a conference funded in part by the NCCAM and convened by the American Society for Microbiology presented evidence that probiotics could also treat urinary tract infections, reduce the recurrence of bladder cancer, and prevent eczema in children.

The research supporting these conclusions is not yet definitive; additional peer-reviewed studies will be needed to prove claims made by scientists... and probiotics manufacturers. Part of the skepticism is due to the fact that the human digestive tract is a vast, complex, interconnected system. It breaks down food into energy and nutrients, hosts ceaseless battles between pathogens and the body's defensive arsenal, and sometimes attacks itself in the form of ulcers, inflammation, and other conditions.

Scientists do not yet fully understand these relationships; thus, the effect of a single element such as probiotics in this system hasn't been fully explored. Moreover, human experiments investigating the effects of probiotics on cancer have so far involved only small numbers of participants; the results are difficult to assess without better controls for other factors. (For example, a 2009 report published in the *Journal of Clinical Gastroenterology* concluded that the human immune system

MEET THE BACTERIA

◆

These microorganisms have been shown to boost health in scientific studies:

STRAIN	BENEFITS	PRODUCTS
Bifidobacterium animalis DN-173 010 (marketing name: Bifidis Regularis)	*Gut health and faster digestion*	Dannon Activia yogurt
Bifidobacterium infantis 356624	*Alleviates symptoms of irritable bowel syndrome*	Procter & Gamble's Align supplement
Bifidobacterium lactis Bb-12	*Helps immune system and digestive health*	Yo-Plus yogurt, Nestle Good Start infant formula
Lactobacillus casei Shirota	*Helps immune system and digestive health*	Yakult fermented dairy drink
Lactobacillus casei DN-114 001 (marketing name: L. casei immunitas)	*Helps immune system; lessens duration of colds and flus in older people*	Dannon's DanActive dairy drink
Lactobacillus GR-1 in combination with **Lactobacillus reuteri**	*Improved vaginal health; helps eradicate vaginal infections*	RepHresh Pro-B and Fem-Dophilus dietary supplements
Lactobacillus reuteri 55730	*Helps treat colic, gingivitis, antibiotic-associated diarrhea*	BioGaia tablets, drops, and lozenges
Saccharomyces boulardii yeast	*Helps prevent and treat antibiotic-associated diarrhea*	Florastor dietary supplement

is "definitely affected by the administration of probiotics." It did not say, however, just *how* useful they were nor which ones were most effective.) Recently yogurt manufacturer Dannon settled a lawsuit that claimed the company overstated the effectiveness of its probiotic foods. (Dannon says it settled the lawsuit to avoid expensive litigation and to focus its efforts instead on products "that provide proven health benefits" to its customers.)

Still, interest in probiotics has been growing rapidly. Americans' spending on probiotic supplements nearly tripled between 1994 and 2003, and between 2007 and 2008 alone, spending on them rose another 16 percent, to $425 million. That figure passed $1 billion in 2009.

Share in the Secret

If you want to take advantage of probiotics, your first task is to change any habits that are destroying your naturally occurring healthy bacteria. These include poor food choices, stress, excessive alcohol consumption, and antibiotics overuse. Next, you want to replenish your friendly bacteria by consuming it in your diet. Probiotic-rich food choices include fermented soybean pastes such as miso and tempeh; yogurt and yogurt drinks like kefir; sauerkraut and many pickles; probiotic soy milk; and other fortified foods. You can also find probiotics in unexpected foods such as certain wines, beers, cottage and other cheeses, and in a popular drink, kombucha, a slightly sour, effervescent fermented tea from Asia. Now sold in health food and gourmet markets, kombucha comes in a wide range of flavors, including cola and ginger.

Just remember that probiotics are living organisms, and like any other living thing, will die if they sit around too long uncared for. Therefore, avoid buying products that aren't fresh, and you must follow the directions on their labels to make sure you are keeping your microscopic allies alive.

You can also take probiotic supplements from a reputable company, such as Ultimate Flora or Source Naturals. Your best bet is a mixture of various flora, including *Lactobacillus acidophilus, Lactobacillus rhamnosus,* and/or some of the *bacidobacterium* strains, such as *bifidum, lactis,* and or *animalis.* Probiotics carry few serious risks, but should be avoided by people who are critically ill or have weakened immune systems.

Also, you need to make sure you are eating the right bacteria, as the health benefits of each strain vary widely within a given bacterium. For

THE YOGURT LONGEVITY MYTH

For many years, television commercials for yogurt featured a group of hardy centenarians living in the Caucasus mountains, plowing fields and walking to markets. According to the ads, the elders owed their health to their yogurt-based diets.

However, it turned out these people were actually much younger than one hundred. They just *looked* old.

The myth of the Caucasians sprang from two factors. One is what's called the nationalist longevity myth: It's common for countries to claim their citizens live to a very old age as a way of promoting their lifestyle. Many nations have done this, including America, where, in 1967, *Time* magazine featured two men who maintained (without proof) that they were each 125 years old. The Soviet Union countered with a Russian named Shirali Mislimov, who said he was nearing 170.

In the 1970 census, more than a hundred thousand people claimed to be more than one hundred years old. But as the Cold War faded, so did the need for the two cultures to fight over which one engendered the oldest citizens, and soon very few people were making such assertions.

The other source of the Caucasus myth was more a matter of self-preservation than nationalism. Many Soviet men doctored their birth certificates to avoid serving in the military.

According to the *Guinness Book of World Records*, about fifty people have been documented to have reached the age of 114; only about twenty of them made it to 115. Two people are verified to have lived past 120, including Jean Calment, the longest-lived person in modern history. Calment (1875–1997) was a Frenchwoman who remembered meeting Vincent van Gogh; she ascribed her longevity to olive oil, which she poured on her food and rubbed into her skin, as well as a daily glass of port wine and about two pounds of chocolate a week.

instance, if a product says it contains *Lactobacillus*, it could be referring to any number of strains including *L. acidophilus*, *L. rhamnosus GG*, *L. casei*, *L. casei* DN-114, or *L. casei* Shirota. In an interview with

The New York Times, Gregor Reid, director of the Canadian Research and Development Center for Probiotics, explained it like this: "To say a product contains *Lactobacillus* is like saying you're bringing George Clooney to a party. It may be the actor, or it may be an eighty-five-year-old guy from Atlanta who just happens to be named George Clooney. With probiotics, there are strain-to-strain differences."

Benefiting from probiotics is about finding a strain or combination of strains that works for you. Regardless of what kinds you consume, you need to maintain steady doses every day for at least a week to see benefits.

Read the instructions that come with your products carefully, and monitor your reaction when you first take them. They can cause mild side effects, such as gas or bloating, while your intestinal microflora balances themselves. Happily, even if you do experience these side effects, they typically pass in about a week.

Running

HELEN KLEIN

After a childhood spent in western Pennsylvania and stints residing in New York City and on Long Island, Helen Klein seemed destined to a pleasant if not particularly unusual life. She stayed home to raise her four children until they went to college, only then returning to work as a nurse at Cleveland's Mount Sinai School of Nursing. Since then she's lived in California, Ohio, and Kentucky, where her husband, Norman (who is fifteen years her junior), did his medical residency and eventually opened a practice.

In 1978, Norman was asked to compete in a ten-mile race. Although he'd never run before, he accepted the challenge—which meant Helen did, too, because the couple does everything together.

Helen was already in good shape, thanks to a powerful lower body and "great quads," which she attributes to an on-the-job workout of lifting heavy patients. But she wasn't aerobically fit, so she trained for ten weeks until she could run the ten miles.

At the time, few women were running competitively. For this race, forty-six men and just four women showed up; Helen, at age fifty-five, was the oldest, and won the trophy for entrants forty and older. Liking the outcome, she decided to run three miles every day to stay fit. And since Norman now wanted to run the Boston Marathon, she trained with him. Eventually, Helen became more than just an occasional marathoner. Today, at 86, she has run 90 marathons, 143 longer races (including 28 hundred-milers), and many eco-challenges (multiday races whose events include adventure sports, from rappelling to white-water rafting).

All told, Helen holds approximately seventy-five world and American records for her age group—including a world record for running across the state of Colorado in five days, ten hours. She's the oldest person ever to complete a hundred-mile trail run and, at age seventy-five, she took on a 145-mile race in the Himalayas. She's finished the Ironman triathlon in Hawaii and a 143-mile stage race across the Peruvian Andes and has broken records in marathon running as recently as 2009.

"I never put a limit on myself because of my age or gender," she says. "If it's in the realm of possibility that I can finish something, I try." Today Helen also devotes time to her nine grandchildren and four great-grandchildren. Other than that, she is actually a laid-back person. "I was raised differently from girls of today. I was raised to be in the background, to be behind the husband and push him up the ladder. We didn't do anything sportswise, growing up. We learned to knit, sew, and cook, sit on the porch and play jacks."

Since she began running, Helen can't recall a day when she's been sick, although she remembers getting the flu rather often as a kid. And she takes no prescription medications. She believes it's the exercise that keeps her well.

But she no longer runs as intensively as she used to: Her husband can run only short races now, although they both still run three to ten miles every morning.

AEROBIC VERSUS ANAEROBIC

◆

Exercise is generally separated into two types of activity: aerobic and anaerobic. The terms refer to different ways the body can make energy—with oxygen or without oxygen. When we're at rest, we have plenty of oxygen to use when we break down carbohydrates and convert them into energy. When we're jogging, say, those muscle cells need more energy, and so we have to breathe harder to take in additional oxygen. Jogging and other types of exercise that make us gulp for breath are aerobic.

Anaerobic exercise is the type of movement, such as lifting a dumbbell, for which our cells need a tremendous amount of energy very quickly. Your biceps' cells can't gather enough oxygen to make all that energy by themselves, so they need to turn carbs into energy without oxygen—a less efficient approach and one that leaves the muscle with a residue called lactic acid. That stuff can sting.

If you have any doubt which type of exercise you're doing, remember this commonly quoted rule: If you're out of breath, it's probably aerobic. If your muscles burn, it's anaerobic.

Helen also runs less these days because she values her privacy. Every time she hits the pavement, the press comes out to watch. "It's difficult to do something well with cameras on you all the time."

Though her children are very active in sports such as cycling and swimming, they don't run. If your mother were Helen Klein, they ask, would you?

The Facts on Running

In the second century A.D., the Greek physician Galen had few tools with which to measure his patients' health. There were no digital heart-rate monitors or stethoscopes, and no one knew how blood circulates or even that there is a connection between germs and disease. But Galen did have gladiators, a parade of bodies put through the most strenuous of physical tests; they allowed the doctor to observe the human body at work.

After years of study, Galen formulated a theory: The body desires movement—and not just the everyday living variety. People need vigor. "The criterion of vigorousness is change of respiration; those movements which do not alter the respiration are not called exercise," he wrote. In other words, movement isn't exercise until you're out of breath.

Today we call that kind of activity *aerobic* exercise.

Down through the centuries, the popularity of exercise has fluctuated, and its forms have changed. However, the concept of exercise as something separate from work is a relatively modern one. The technological and social advances that brought about the phenomenon of leisure time meant that an increasing number of people were no longer forced to exercise (as in manual labor) to make a living. Now they wanted to exercise to promote relaxation and enhance fitness. By the turn of the twentieth century, many well-known Americans were touting exercise's benefits, including President Teddy Roosevelt, who claimed that his commitment to fitness was the bridge between his sickly youth and his rugged Rough Rider days.

> "A MAN'S HEALTH *can be judged by which he takes two at a time—pills or stairs."*
>
> ~JOAN WELSH

But medicine lagged behind society; nearly two millennia passed before scientists began to explore Galen's theories. According to the U.S. Department of Health and Human Services (HHS), one third of the men drafted to serve in the American Expeditionary Force in World War I were found to be physically unfit. Wellness now became a matter of national defense, and research dollars flowed. For example, between 1924 and 1946, Harvard's Fatigue Laboratory continually tested the effects of work and strain on the human body, and by the 1950s, the American Medical Association was investigating the links between exercise and fitness, while fitness pioneer Jack LaLanne was swimming across San Francisco Bay to promote exercise. LaLanne was also the first fitness guru to effectively use the new medium of television to popularize working out. Fitness had arrived in the public consciousness.

Scientists have continued to study and praise the effects of exercise. A 2002 metastudy published by HHS titled "Physical Activity Fundamental to Preventing Disease" listed the health benefits of exercise (defined as thirty minutes of moderate activity five days a week): reducing the risk of developing or dying from heart disease and of developing diabetes, high blood pressure, colon cancer, and breast cancer; driving down already dangerously high blood pressure; and easing depression and anxiety while promoting psychological well-being.

Study after study has confirmed these findings. Take, for example, diabetes: In the landmark Diabetes Prevention Program study, published in 2002 by the *New England Journal of Medicine*, researchers found that participants who maintained a healthy diet and exercise routine reduced their risk of developing diabetes by 58 percent, while the group that took an antidiabetic drug reduced their risk by only 31 percent.

Exercise has not only been shown to help prevent diabetes but can also help diabetics overcome the effects of the disease. In a study published in *Diabetic Care* in 2009, an exercise program including both aerobic and anaerobic (strength training) elements was shown to improve the body's capacity to control glucose (blood sugar) levels in participants who had already developed type 2 diabetes.

Researchers are also finding links between exercise and the immune system, corroborating the long held belief among runners, such as Helen Klein, that their activity helps them ward off infectious illnesses. Admittedly, this area of study is still relatively new. According to the *International Journal of Sports Medicine,* of the 629 papers published on exercise and immunity in the twentieth century, 378 were written in its last decade. (And because of the ethical implications of manipulating human immunity, most of the earlier data come from experiments using mice.)

Exercise has also recently been shown to mitigate the effects of chronic stress. Stress has physiological implications that aggravate the

JEREMY MORRIS TAKES A BUS

For millennia, people have believed that good health is related to exercise, but no one knew exactly why. The first exercise that proved its benefit through scientific study wasn't running or aerobics or even walking. It was climbing stairs on a double-decker bus.

In the late 1940s, British epidemiologist Jeremy Morris began examining the heart-attack rates of the public bus staff to see if there was a difference in rates between the sedentary drivers, who seldom moved, and the conductors, who continually climbed the stairs. There was: Morris's data revealed that the conductors suffered fewer than half the heart attacks that drivers did.

Morris's studies of workers in other professions found corroborating evidence that exercise played a role

in better health. For example, postal workers who were active, spending their days delivering mail, had a lower risk of heart attack than those with an office desk job.

Morris's work formed the basis of today's understanding of the relationship between exercise and cardiovascular disease. He received many awards, including the first International Olympic Committee Medal in sports science in 1972. Not surprisingly, Morris himself exercised throughout his life, swimming, riding a stationary bike, or walking for at least half an hour nearly every day until well into his nineties. He died in 2009, just before his hundredth birthday, of pneumonia and kidney failure. His heart, however, was still in good shape.

conditions of people already at risk for heart disease because it places more—and more constant—strain on the heart by increasing blood pressure. That's one reason the Mayo Clinic recommends physical activity to counter the negative effects of stress, citing the meditative state it induces, along with its antidepression effects and the boost in endorphins it generates.

As always, the secret must be handled sensibly. Because of these pleasurable effects, and because so many of the healthful benefits of exercise seem to be dose-dependent, some people tend to take exercise too far. And with overexertion, exercise-induced stimulation of the immune system can turn into immune *suppression.*

The cellular mechanics involved in exercise's effects on immunity are still being explored, but we do know that exercise affects the quantity and functioning of several types of white blood cells that comprise our immune defenses. Recent studies confirm that, as a 1997 article in the *Journal of Applied Physiology* put it, there is "growing evidence that, for several hours subsequent to heavy exertion, several components of . . . the immune system exhibit suppressed function." This suppression, the study showed, led to measurably higher rates of upper-respiratory tract infections in athletes during training, and for one to two weeks following their races.

And running may be as bad for your bones as it is good for your heart. A British study of women runners, for example, found that running ten extra kilometers per week corresponded with almost 2 percent lower bone density. However, the researchers suggest that this result may be because women who commit to vigorous training also often restrict their diets, thus risking a nutritional deficiency.

The bottom line: Running is good for you because it's strenuous. But because it's strenuous, you have to run intelligently.

Share in the Secret

Start running. Few exercise routines are begun more easily. Although it's always a good idea to talk to your doctor first, the odds are you'll be fine—but check in nonetheless. You just need running shoes, weather-appropriate clothes, and a place to do it.

There is no compelling safety reason to spend a great deal of money on good running shoes, but it is possible to buy more comfort. Once you start running longer distances, you'll begin to understand what some of those ads for premium shoes mean by claiming to counteract heat and humidity. (However, some people are forgoing shoes altogether, on the theory that our feet and legs are exceptionally good at dispersing shock and that running without shoes promotes better running form by keeping runners off their heels, enforcing a forward falling motion. There are no conclusive studies on barefoot running, but many runners swear that it has cured their chronic aches and injuries. For safety's sake, barefooters run only on special indoor tracks.

Once you have your shoes (and your iPod, your water bottle, your pedometer, your headband, and so on), how far are you actually supposed to run? Few of us are natural runners like Helen Klein. As a general rule, the CDC recommends that an adult get seventy-five minutes of vigorous aerobic activity each week. Whether or not you want to accomplish that task in two, three, four, or seven days is up to you. The word *vigorous* hasn't changed much since Galen used it, but can mean very different things to different people.

If you are just starting out, you can alternate walking and running. Each session, try running more and walking less. You'll find your own running pace, so it's important to start out by measuring minutes and not miles. (It's going to feel a lot harder than those people who hit the pavement at six A.M. make it look.) Don't worry—it gets easier within a few weeks. It'll also get more rewarding. Running websites recommend that you start out by fitting running into your errands: If you end up at the grocery store, it'll feel like you got something done and didn't just run around in a circle.

Start slowly, make it a routine, and learn to enjoy that runner's high—the release of endorphins and other happy-making chemicals in the brain that results from strenuous exercise. But monitor your body. Not everyone will profit from running, and a multitude of injuries, from fractured hip joints to pulled hamstrings to arch pain, are all possible. Oddly, the runner's high can be present even when you may be hurting yourself; the rush is that pleasurable. After each run, check your body to make sure that, as much as you want to run, it wants to also.

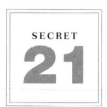
Spirituality

JOHN JOSEPH

When John Joseph, aka John Joseph McGowan, aka Bloodclot, performs on stage with his band, audience members show their enthusiasm by stage-diving (jumping up onstage, then throwing themselves back into the audience). Meanwhile, John dashes about like a whirling dervish—spinning, jumping, and backflipping. Pretty good for a forty-six-year old.

"People tell me it's the most intense, energetic shit they've ever seen—especially given my age. Everyone I know playing music is all about their bad knees, their bad joints, their bad back. I'm still in it."

John grew up on the streets of New York City, tossed around from one foster home to another, beaten and abused by parents and the system alike. By fourteen, he was dealing drugs; by sixteen, he'd wound up in a juvenile correctional facility. A few years later, he joined the

CHRISTIAN SCIENCE

◆

There are few more prominent examples of the intersection of spirituality and health than the First Church of Christ, Scientist, a religious denomination that promotes prayer to cure physical, mental, and emotional ailments.

The church was founded in 1879 by an American woman named Mary Baker Eddy. Chronically ill from a young age, Eddy spent much of her life researching homeopathic medicine and looking for spiritual guidance in the Bible. After a fall on an icy sidewalk left her in critical condition, she claimed to have healed herself by reading an account of Jesus' healing power. Nine years after the fall, she published the bestselling book *Science and Health with Key to the Scriptures,* which explains the "science" behind her religious healing method.

The religion is probably most famous for its continued reliance upon prayer to heal the body; its practitioners do not believe in Western medicine and they shun doctors. Church doctrine declares:

"Christian Science treatment is the application of spiritual principles— who and what God is and what that means for each individual—to the specifics of any given situation. These spiritual principles, applied, have a tangible effect—restored relationships, financial well-being, physical healing, and so on." This practice has recently received much negative press, as several high-profile cases have documented the deaths of children whose Christian Scientist parents withheld medical intervention, particularly the 2008 case of an eleven-year-old Wisconsin girl who wasn't given care for her treatable diabetes.

When Eddy was eighty-seven, Joseph Pulitzer's tabloid newspaper, the *New York World,* attacked her and her belief system, and Eddy responded by creating the *Christian Science Monitor,* a secular news publication that aimed "to injure no man but to bless all mankind." The *Monitor* went on to win dozens of Overseas Press Club awards and, ironically, seven Pulitzer Prizes.

Navy; a few months after that, he went AWOL. Eventually he spent a few months in a military prison.

Drug-addicted, ambitionless, angry, empty, John barely survived the 1970s. Roaming New York's dark streets left him with little regard for human life, and he assumed he'd die young, like his cohorts. Instead, he got his life together by becoming lead singer of the Cro-Mags, a hardcore punk band. Around the same time, he met the Bad Brains, punk rockers who blew him away musically... and spiritually. The band's members were Rastafarians, which got John thinking about his life in new terms.

"As a result of all I went through as a kid, sure, I found myself questioning whether God exists. Then I finally started becoming interested in something beyond myself."

John became the Bad Brains' roadie/security guard. Along the way, he read countless books on religion, later spending two years at an ashram, an Indian spiritual retreat. During this pilgrimage, his life shifted from one of averting disaster to one of seeking spirituality. He shaved his head, rose before dawn to meditate each day, and focused on restoring his health, which had been unstable and drug-addled. His overall well-being improved to the point where, despite a grueling schedule of concerts around the United States and Europe, he's never ill.

"I'm not getting up at four in the morning anymore, but I still chant every day. It's part of what keeps me healthy. The Vedas [sacred texts of Hinduism] say the three causes of disease are overanxiety, uncleanness, and overeating. So I do breathing exercises, daily yoga, eat organic vegan, and do weight and resistance training. You have to train like crazy to absorb all of this."

When his band goes on tour, given the late hours, the tough gigs, and the coughing and sneezing at close quarters, most of the band returns home sick. John doesn't. "The spiritual path saved me. That's not some cliché. Everyone else I knew from the streets is in jail or dead. If the divine hadn't intervened, I wouldn't be here."

The Facts on Spirituality

Lourdes, a small town in southern France, has a native population of only fifteen thousand, but it hosts as many as five million visitors a year.

Most of them come seeking the town's waters, purported for a century and a half to heal the sick.

The legend of Lourdes springs from a day in February 1858 when a fourteen-year-old girl named Bernadette Soubirous claimed that a beautiful woman, "lovelier than I have ever seen," appeared before her in the Grotto of Massabielle, a fetid spot that had served as a local pasture and garbage dump. People came to believe that the beautiful woman, whom Bernadette saw about eighteen times, was the Virgin Mary.

A shrine was eventually built, and since then has attracted approximately 200 million people because it quickly became famous for curing scores of people, even those with chronically incurable conditions. The Roman Catholic Church, which oversees the site, has recognized sixty-seven official "miraculous healings" there—from cancer cures to reversals of paralysis. The Church claims there could be no explanation other than divine intervention.

Are the miracles at Lourdes real? Can faith keep us healthy? Can spirituality improve your chances for surviving a critical illness? These questions, once met with a high degree of skepticism, are currently being investigated. However, health and religion have actually been intertwined since the beginning of written history—and probably earlier.

Historians believe medicine was first practiced by shamans and priest-healers tens of thousands of years ago. These healers used their connection to the spirit world to treat their fellow tribespeople here in the material world; in various indigenous cultures around the world, shamans still practice this kind of medicine.

The earliest known medical texts come from the ancient civilization of Mesopotamia, where wellness was associated with harmony, the seasons, and the natural cycles of life—all considered the realms of the gods. The ancients believed that illness represented a break from these natural forces and that health could be restored by reconnecting with them; the modern symbol of the medical profession—two snakes coiling around a staff—derives from this belief. Known as the caduceus, the image depicts Ningishzida, the Sumerian god of nature and fertility.

Similarly, in Egyptian mythology, illness was seen as an imbalance of cosmic and earthly forces. The Greeks (and later the Romans) deified Asclepius, son of Apollo and god of medicine, who also oversaw healing and health care. Good health was synonymous with a good relationship with the gods.

After the fall of Rome, Christian monks became the guardians of the ancient world's health secrets, incorporating pagan remedies where useful and helping to preserve ancient pharmacology. Progress, however, was scant; until the seventeenth century, the most revered texts in medical circles were still those written by Galen, the second-century Greek physician. Then, with the development of modern scientific principles, medicine began to veer away from its part-Classical, part-spiritual approach toward the evidence-based Western model still extant today, one that emphasizes research, controlled blind studies, pharmacology, and specialization.

Yet despite its spectacular advances, modern medical science can still be bested by chronic diseases and mysterious ailments. At such times, evidence increasingly shows that faith can offer more than solace: It can actually assist the healing process.

Among the scores of corroborating reports for this view are a 1998 Duke University study, funded by the National Institute of Mental Health, that found the degree of religious faith among the disabled and chronically ill had a measurable effect on the speed of their recovery from depression. A 2000 study published by the *Journal of Substance Abuse Treatment* that said "higher levels of religious faith and spirituality were associated with a more optimistic life orientation, greater perceived social support, higher resilience to stress, and lower levels of anxiety." And a U.S. Office of Technology Assessment review of a decade's worth of articles published in the *Journal of Family Practice* that found 83 percent of studies on religiosity showed a positive correlation with physical health. A similar survey of two major psychiatric journals revealed that 92 percent of the studies reported mental-health benefits from participating in organized religion.

Spiritual people also seem to have better-functioning immune systems, according to a 1997 study published in the *Journal of Psychiatry in Medicine*. Researchers compared the immune cells of regular churchgoers with those of people who didn't attend, finding that the irreligious were twice as likely to have elevated levels of interleukin-6, an immune protein associated with a wide variety of age-related diseases.

One of the most prominent studies in this area investigated the power of prayer. Conducted in 1988 by Dr. Randolph Byrd at San Francisco General Hospital's cardiac unit, it divided 393 patients into two groups: One was the object of prayers from strangers, the other received no prayers. (The patients themselves did not know to which group they belonged.) Results showed that the patients who received no prayers were nearly twice as likely to suffer complications of their disease as those who did.

Despite the myriad studies showing a positive relationship between spirituality and health, many others show none at all. Perhaps the earliest such research appeared in the 1870s, when Charles Darwin's cousin, Francis Galton, decided to test the power of prayer. Galton realized that the most prayed-for people in England at the time were the royal family. So if prayer worked, shouldn't the members of the royal family live long and healthy lives? Far from proving that, his statistical analysis showed they actually died sooner than the average Englishman.

And many recent studies (conducted after Byrd's prayer investigation) have likewise found no conclusive evidence that patients for whom prayers were said showed a positive health reaction. Also, some of the studies linking spirituality to good health have been dismissed for methodological flaws. Richard P. Sloan, PhD, professor of behavioral medicine at Columbia University, points out the tricky ethics involved in prescribing religion, saying, "By suggesting to patients that religious activity is associated with better health, you also imply the converse— that poor health is a product of insufficient religious activity."

Physicians aren't the only critics on this issue. An article by Richard Sloan published in the June 2000 issue of the *New England*

Journal of Medicine was coauthored by seven religious leaders, including
Protestants, Buddhists, and Catholics; in it, Sloan says the media are
partly to blame for the hype by giving prominent press coverage only
to studies showing a positive impact of religion on health and ignoring
evidence to the contrary.

More troublesome are the bitter
debates over the place of spirituality and
religion in modern health care. The clashes
over abortion and euthanasia rend society,
creating factions that can find no common
ground. And recent cases of parents who
withheld medical treatment from their
children for religious reasons have made
headlines when the child died. Although most states have laws allowing
some religious exemptions for parents who balk at conventional medicine
for their sick children, none allows parents to substitute spirituality for
medical care for serious conditions.

> "SO MANY PEOPLE *spend their
> health gaining wealth, and
> then have to spend their wealth
> to regain their health."*
> ~A. J. REB MATERI, AUTHOR

There is no area of health more controversial than the proper place
of spirituality within its confines. All of us must decide how to balance
our belief systems and our health care needs. Yet keeping an open
mind seems to offer more options than otherwise. Those who came to
the shrine at Lourdes ill and left healthy, and John Joseph, who firmly
believes that faith is his secret to health, attest to that.

Share in the Secret

How to become spiritual? This is probably the hardest of all the secrets
to share. It requires a Kierkegaardian leap of faith: leaving behind your
rational self for a world where faith rather than logic rules. Furthermore,
the range of spiritual practices available today is enormous; different
people find spirituality in different places. Many practice it through the
observance of an organized religion and the belief in a higher power.
Others find it in nature, music, or other forms of secular community.

Becoming more spiritual seems like a vague and daunting task, but people have been trying to do it, and succeeding, for eons. Here is some advice from one of the world's leading experts on spirituality, theologian and psychotherapist Thomas Moore, whose many bestselling books include *Care of the Soul, Dark Nights of the Soul, and Care of the Soul in Medicine*:

One of the greatest dangers to health is to live unconsciously, absorbing the ideas and values of the culture, especially through mass media. Living that way, you are not fully alive and never get to enjoy your individuality. You may well get depressed easily and feel like a wanderer, not entirely sure who you are and what to do.

The spiritual traditions of the world offer several ways to develop and intensify your spiritual existence. The first step they all recommend is to "wake up." Once you begin to wake up to the possibilities of your life, you can begin to focus on a few specific items that will keep you spiritually awake and alive:

NATURE

Spending time in nature, observing its mysteries and curious forms of vitality, takes you out of yourself and puts you in touch with the liveliness of the world you inhabit. This connection is the basis of a spiritual life. You don't have to travel far but can find what you need in a park or garden or small river.

MEDITATION

Your meditation doesn't have to be formal or lengthy. Walk thoughtfully, sit reflectively, especially in those in-between moments of everyday life—waiting for a train or bus, walking from one place to another.

ART

Most art has a spiritual quality, even if it's only a still life helping you contemplate ordinary things. But you can look for good spiritual art, too. You can have a statue of the Buddha, Jesus, Quan Yin, the Virgin Mary, African spirits, Northwest America totems—all of these can keep your focus on the mysteries of life.

PRAYER

A Renaissance theologian once said that religion is as natural to a human being as barking is to a dog. I'd say the same about prayer. You can always say a quiet, inner prayer asking for what you need, praising what you see, thanking the source of life for what you have.

SPIRITUAL READING

This is not reading for information, but slow and reflective reading for inspiration and contemplation. You can read poetry or fiction or nature writing or spiritual ideas— read them off and on throughout the day; then reflect upon what you have read.

These few items offer a beginning. The list could go on. Today you can learn these things from basic spiritual traditional and sacred texts: the Tao Te Ching, the Buddhist Heart Sutra, the Gospels, the Psalms, Sufi poems, Native American prayers. Borrow from unfamiliar traditions and go deeper into the one you know best. Your spirit will rise like yeast, and your sense of self will expand.

The connections between the mind, body, and spirit are just beginning to be understood. In order to learn their secrets, researchers are overcoming hundreds of years of mutual skepticism between Western medical and religious traditions. In the end, the connection between spirituality and health may lie less in what people believe and more in how strongly they believe it. As Herbert Benson, MD, of Harvard Medical School said in a 1998 interview with the *Shambhala Sun*: "If you believe, in one extreme, in a sugar pill, that belief can help you heal. It almost doesn't matter what you believe in, in a religious belief, in your doctor, in nature itself. We all have a belief in something and we have to tie in the power of the body to heal with what we believe in, which may be different from person to person."

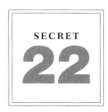

Stresslessness

SUSAN SMITH JONES

"I don't let stress into my life, even when it tries really, really hard to enter it," says Susan Smith Jones. For example, one recent Sunday she was driving on a congested Southern California freeway when her engine began emitting small puffs of smoke. Cruising in the fast lane, she tried to pull over, but made it only as far as the middle lane before the car stopped dead. She was now stuck on a packed freeway in sweltering, 100-plus-degree heat, surrounded by yelling, honking motorists and vulnerable to getting hit from behind and causing a major pile-up—as well as dying right then and there.

After a few moments of panic, she took several deep breaths, indulged in a moment of prayer, and kept herself serene until another motorist pulled up and offered to help. He called the police, and soon enough her car was being pushed to the nearest exit ramp. Susan 1, stress, 0.

A native Californian with three degrees from UCLA, Susan has made a career of stresslessness. She's taught health and fitness, written twenty books (including her newest, *The Joy Factor*) and eight hundred magazine articles, and she has given talks throughout the world on holistic health and stress reduction.

Her devotion to a natural, stress-free life began when she was a teenager and fell ill. Her doctor then gave her a prescription for allergy medicine. But Susan's grandmother Fritzie, who had grown up in Denmark, had other ideas. She offered to teach Susan the natural home remedies she had learned as a child and had practiced ever since. As a result of working with Fritzie for seven years as her assistant and protégé, Susan became a holistic healer and an expert on relaxation.

One of Fritzie's lessons was to treat the body with loving care to support its own inherent healing ability, and a primary form of that care is stress management. "Two thirds of all visits to the doctor are due to stress-related ailments," Susan claims, "and 80 to 90 percent of all diseases are stress related. If you control your stress, you control your immunity to disease."

So it seems. Susan has never taken medication and doesn't even keep aspirin in her home. Nor has she had a cold or a flu in twenty-five years.

For Susan, self-care means a stressless daily life. Believing that the first forty minutes of the morning set the tone for the entire day, she rises at four A.M. to meditate—eyes closed, breathing slowly and deeply and yes, unlike most people, she thinks rising at that hour is pure joy. Then she squeezes fresh juice using organic produce picked from her garden (gardening is another way to reduce stress), takes an early-morning hike in the Santa Monica mountains, and eats a substantial vegan breakfast. She writes or reads till lunchtime, when she eats a salad or a sandwich, typically some type of raw food on whole-grain bread. Whatever the meal, it's likely to include sprouts, which she literally grows all over her kitchen. Always in the background is relaxing music or nature sounds.

MOSES SUPPOSES NEUROSES ARE ROSES

◆

Please don't get stressed out and neurotic about the advice in this book—especially if you're male. A recent study from researchers at Purdue and Boston universities, published in *Psychological Science*, looked at more than 1,700 men aged forty to ninety-one to see how neurotic men's health fared over thirty years (neurotic being defined as a someone who worries too much, easily lapses into depression, and reacts negatively to stress). The authors contrasted such men with other men who weren't as neurotic, and by the end of the study, they found that only half of the former group were alive, compared to 75 to 85 percent of the other group. According to the report, even a small increase in the level of the subject's neuroticism during the period of the study resulted in a 40 percent increase in death compared to the less neurotic.

In the afternoon, Susan sees clients in her private practice. Later she might join a friend for a quiet dinner, or read. She turns in around eight P.M., after another meditation session. "I believe that we always attract to ourselves the equivalent of what we think, believe, feel, say, and do, so I continually monitor my thoughts and feelings and make sure that I'm always giving out what I desire back. To bring more peace into our lives, we must choose to live more peacefully—day to day. I strive daily to embrace a peaceful, stressless lifestyle."

Susan thinks attitude is the mind's paintbrush—color hers stressless.

The Facts on Stress

Stress (as we think of it today) has been around for only about sixty years. In the nineteenth century, the concept referred not to human physiology but to the application of pressure to metal. Back then, people feeling overburdened with life's problems were said to suffer a deficiency in their "nerve force."

Things began to change in 1869, when New York neurologist George Beard coined the term *neurasthenia* for a nervous-system malfunction brought on by stressors such as harsh climates, overwork, and what even then was considered the fast pace of modern life. His ideas remained popular until the early twentieth century, falling out of favor until revived by the work of two men. The first was Harvard physiologist Walter B. Cannon, who in 1929 coined the term *fight or flight* for the biological processes stimulated in mammals whenever we're in imminent danger. The increased respiration, muscle tension, and adrenalin rush enhance our ability either to fight or to flee a threat. Cannon concluded that the prevalence of stressors in modern life was so great that the human body's innate responses were being chronically stimulated, causing us harm rather than preventing us from being eaten.

Cannon's work focused on the effect of strong emotional experiences, but stopped short of developing a more general theory of stress and its effects. This task fell to Vienna-born Canadian physician and biochemist Hans Selye, who in the 1950s used the word *stress* to mean the response people have to day-to-day, high-pressure situations.

When his work was slow to catch on within the medical community, Selye publicized it through articles in popular magazines, such as *Reader's Digest*; by the 1970s, the concept of stress was part of our modern vocabulary. Selye also promoted the idea that certain people were particularly vulnerable to stress. Dubbed type A personalities, these people are highly aggressive individuals whose disposition makes them more vulnerable to heart attack and other illnesses.

Selye's work provoked an enormous amount of research, demonstrating the ill effects of stress on human health. Today, if you look up "stress" on Amazon.com, you'll find thirty thousand references to books. Search "stress and health" on Google and you'll get more than a hundred thousand results. Universities offer courses on the topic, hundreds of academic seminars on the subject are presented yearly, and thousands of workshops are offered by so-called experts in stress and health management across the country.

All the research indicates that stress can kill. According to a 2003 study from the University of Wales College of Medicine published in *Psychosomatic Medicine,* people with type A personalities are much more likely to have heart attacks than others: "The data show Type A is a strong predictor of when incident coronary heart disease (or coronary event) will occur rather than if it will occur." Research from Duke University showed that stress damages the immune system and the heart; investigators found that 27 percent of those who responded adversely to mental stress testing later suffered heart problems. Other studies suggest that stress conditions increase the chances of contracting bacterial infections such as tuberculosis and certain streptococcal diseases; you're more likely to catch a cold due to lowered immune system response.

In fact, the list of conditions that stress has been shown to precipitate is frighteningly extensive, including sleeplessness, lack of energy, backaches, diarrhea, constipation, depression, bloating, cramping, changes in appetite, listlessness, irritability, likeliness to develop asthma, rashes, hives, irritable bowel syndrome, diabetes, and high blood pressure.

Stress is certainly taking a toll on society as a whole. In England, where it has become the most common excuse for taking time off work, more than 13 million workdays a year are now said to be lost to stress-related health problems.

Still, there are those who think that efforts to defeat stress are unnecessary, that we need to maintain the fight-or-flight response lest we lose the ability to jump out of the way of a moving bus or evade a mugger. If we overly dampen our stress response, we lose our ability to perform well in difficult situations. Stress can be energizing as well as enervating, motivating us to work harder and perform better. It can also stimulate the memory and bring excitement to life.

Others go further, calling the dream of ridding our lives of stress an unhealthy preoccupation: As editor and writer Mick Hume said in

YOUNG STRESS

◆

According to a Stress in America Survey conducted in 2009 by Harris Interactive on behalf of the American Psychological Association, stress is a top health concern for American teens between ninth and twelfth grade. The study suggested that the stress had serious long-term health implications if the kids didn't learn to manage it early.

Their parents, however, don't seem to realize there's a problem. Teens were much more likely than their parents to say that their stress had increased in the past year. Nearly half of young people aged thirteen to seventeen said they worried more this year than last, but only 28 percent of their parents believed their teen's stress had increased.

The Times of London: "The depressing obsession with work stress is symptomatic of a culture that prefers to define the human condition by vulnerability rather than resilience. The 'happiness' that the stress industry seeks for us seems to be a sort of lobotomized existence in a disinfected bubble with soothing piped music. Some of us, however, would rather live in a state of creative stress than of gormless serenity. A stress-free life sounds like a living death."

Share in the Secret

If you believe your health would benefit from reduced stress, you can find plenty of options if you open your wallet wide enough. Scented lotions, aromatherapy candles, stress-management books and music, guided-imagery CDs, bath products, electronic massagers, cushy chairs, herbs, room ionizers, and the new soft drink Drank—all are marketed as stress busters. As Mick Hume suggests, these products are at the core of the booming stress industry. Americans spent an estimated $14 billion fighting stress in 2009, according to Market Data, up $3 billion from the previous year.

But if spending money on stress relief will cause you, well, stress, other solutions are cost-free. Susan Smith Jones, whose newest book is called *The Joy Factor*, offers seven suggestions:

1. Get moving. Exercise is one of the best ways to reduce stress. At the University of Southern California, researchers had patients take a vigorous walk around a track, and found this one simple routine reduced the level of tension in their bodies by 20 percent.

2. Meditate and breathe deeply. Your first 40 minutes in the morning set the tone for your day. Combined with breath work, meditation can balance the flow of stress hormones.

3. Eat a diet that takes stress off your digestive system. That means seven servings of colorful fruits and vegetables a day.

4. Keep your body hydrated. We need to maintain proper fluid balance to support our brain function and our kidneys' ability to rid the body of waste and toxins.

5. Get enough sleep. Six or fewer hours of a sleep a night leaves you irritable and stupid. It also subtracts from your life span and adds pounds—talk about stressful!

6. Laugh. Laughter releases endorphins in the body that act as natural stress busters, and it gives the heart muscle a good workout.

7. Cultivate an "attitude of gratitude." Susan's grandmother Fritzie told her to live thankfully each and every day—first and foremost by appreciating the beauty of nature: the sky, the trees, the animals. Keep a vase of fresh flowers in your bedroom, she recommended, so you can see them before going to sleep at night and first thing in the morning—even if it's just one rose. To keep that attitude constant, Fritzie also encouraged Susan to write down in a gratitude journal at least three things for which she was grateful just before bed, and to think about those things as she fell asleep.

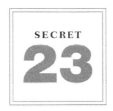

Stretching

DR. ROBERT FULFORD

I n his bestselling book *Spontaneous Healing,* Dr. Andrew Weil devotes a chapter to his mentor, Dr. Robert Fulford. Weil, a traditionally trained physician who's one of the world's most renowned experts on alternative medicine, spent years searching for the world's greatest healer, traveling on all five continents from the Himalayas to the Amazon. He surprised himself when his search uncovered Dr. Fulford, then an octogenarian, near his own home in Arizona.

Dr. Fulford, an MD as well as a DO (doctor of osteopathy), was interested in many different medical therapies. Whenever he found anything efficacious, he would add it to the treatments offered in his practice, no matter what anyone else thought. Due perhaps to this eclectic approach, Dr. Fulford became internationally famous for his ability to heal people on whom conventional doctors had given up.

Dr. Weil's book discusses some of these cases, prompting him to write, "The medicine I saw Dr. Fulford practice was the kind of medicine I had longed for during my years of clinical training and my years of wandering."

Dr. Fulford spent his entire adult life searching for new ways to heal people. He recalled that when he first became interested in alternative medical treatments in the 1930s and '40s, other doctors would walk by his office making duck sounds: "Quack, quack!" Feelings hurt, he persevered, adopting any new theory he felt could be useful, from acupressure to energy medicine.

The quest for new ideas was grounded in Dr. Fulford's basic tenets of health:

1. The body wants to be healthy.

2. Healing is a natural power.

3. The body is a whole, and all its parts are connected.

4. Mind and body are one.

5. The beliefs of practitioners strongly influence the healing powers of patients.

Dr. Fulford believed that the surest way to health was to stimulate the life force that exists within all of us, a force that can be blunted by anything from trauma to illness to poor breathing habits. The best way to stimulate that force, he claimed, was seeing a practitioner like him, who could, among other things, manipulate the patient's body with his or her hands to improve energy flow.

Even in his nineties, Dr. Fulford scoured the medical literature, updated his knowledge base, and continued to see patients. His one concession to age was that he could heal only children; he felt it draining to work with adults, whose energy levels he found too overwhelming to correct.

ARE COLDS OUR FRIENDS?

◆

For the most part, this book offers suggestions for avoiding illness. Always a contrarian, Dr. Fulford had a different view: He believed that an occasional cold could be beneficial. A cold, he said, allowed the body to expel all kinds of noxious substances of which it normally couldn't rid itself. In this view, the mucus from coughs and sneezes is like the outfall of a raging sewer, helping to wash out the detritus our body has no other way to eliminate.

A fever, too, has its advantages, according to Dr. Fulford, who discouraged patients from taking medicine to lower one. He had been schooled to believe the opposite—that we should "encourage the body to react to whatever was trying to manifest itself by developing a fever."

Fulford's fever philosophy has a scientific basis. The body continually burns up waste materials in the form of cells that are constantly dying and being replaced by new ones. If these dead cells aren't able to leave the body in a consistent way, they'll accumulate in large numbers. A fever may be the body's way of incinerating the dead cells and restoring the disposal process.

Thus it's possible a fever is exactly what your body needs—unless your temperature exceeds 103 degrees. In that case, the body is sending a danger signal, one that needs to be addressed by conventional medicine.

Seldom ill throughout his own life, Dr. Fulford was healthier than most people half his age. One of the reasons, he claimed, was a set of stretching exercises he developed with fellow osteopath Dr. Richard Koss. In the absence of hands-on osteopathic treatment, he believed these exercises were the key to staying healthy.

The Facts on Stretching

There is no medical evidence to support Dr. Fulford's claims for his exercises. Controlled studies examining the health benefits of these stretches have never been undertaken, although there is plenty of

OSTEOPATHY

In the late 1800s, Andrew Taylor Still was a troubled man. As a licensed medical doctor, he had seen the horrors of the American Civil War and also watched three of his children die from spinal meningitis. These and other experiences caused him to doubt prevailing medical theories. His response was to create his own medical system, called osteopathy. Emphasizing a "whole person" approach to medicine, it specifically focused on the musculoskeletal system. Still founded the American School of Osteopathy in Kirksville, Missouri, in 1892, and the discipline has since grown to encompass twenty schools with approximately 44,000 accredited practitioners in America, and is growing in popularity around the world as well. DOs have full practice rights in forty-four countries, from Finland to Argentina. Great Britain, where DOs recently gained full practice rights, is now home to over 4,000 of them. Be careful, however—osteopathy is practiced differently in different countries.

DOs believe that the body has an innate ability to heal itself and their job is to promote this ability. Their whole-person approach to healing emphasizes the treatment of the body as an entire system, as opposed to

evidence that stretching per se can be beneficial for muscles and also relieve tension. From an anecdotal perspective, however, much evidence exists. Dr. Fulford recommended these exercises to his patients for more than twenty-five years and reported excellent results. He also did them himself and was seldom, if ever, ill until a few weeks before his death of natural causes at the age of ninety-two.

I first met Dr. Fulford when, at age eighty-eight, he decided to write a book on which he asked me to collaborate. (The book, *Dr. Fulford's Touch of Life,* was published in 1996.) While I was working with him at his home in rural Ohio (he had moved from Arizona back to his native state very late in life), young patients would arrive from all over the country with parents who were both hopeful and in awe of Dr. Fulford.

THE SECRETS OF PEOPLE WHO NEVER GET SICK

176

fighting isolated symptoms; hence the emphasis on the musculoskeletal system. Composing about two thirds of the body's mass, bones and muscles play an integral part in overall well-being. DOs believe that ensuring that bones, muscles, and nerves are functioning properly promotes good health in the rest of the body.

In America, DOs often practice osteopathic manipulative medicine, a form of physical therapy aimed at improving the function of the musculoskeletal system. Although it has been proven to be an effective treatment for lower back and spinal pain in a number of studies, scientific proof for its efficacy in other areas is scant. "I'll freely admit that once you get outside of back disorders and start looking at efficacy in such things as asthma, for instance, the data are not nearly as solid," said Dr. Douglas Wood, former president of the American Association of Colleges of Osteopathic Medicine, in an interview with *The New York Times*.

However, many doctors of osteopathy are also certified allopathic, or conventional Western, physicians who use osteopathy as a complementary form of treatment. For this reason, osteopaths, who for most of the twentieth century were treated as second-class citizens by allopaths, are now working side by side with them in hospitals and clinics.

"Do you see that young woman?" he asked me once. "Her doctors didn't think they could help her, so they asked me to take over. Six months later she's doing great."

Another time a young couple took me aside and explained to me that their doctor had told them that their son would be in pain for the rest of his life due to severe back injuries suffered in a car accident. After just three months of seeing Dr. Fulford, he was pain-free. "We don't understand what's going on," the couple told me, "but we don't care. It's working."

As Dr. Weil writes, "Dr. Fulford did not succeed with everyone, but he had a higher percentage of successful outcomes than any other practitioner I have met."

Share in the Secret

Dr. Fulford's exercises were designed for people of all ages, and they can be done at home or in the office—wherever there's a chair and a wall.

EXERCISE 1

Stand with your feet spread shoulder-width apart. Extend your arms to your sides at approximately shoulder height. Your left palm should face upward and your right downward. Try to stand in this position for a full ten minutes. When you get to the point that you're too tired to hold your arms up any longer, still keeping them straight, slowly raise them above your head without allowing them to come forward. Then lower them.

If this exercise is too demanding, try it while sitting on a couch.

EXERCISE 2

Sitting down, breathe in and out rapidly, imitating the motion of an automobile piston. Take the breath in, and then blow it out right away. Quickly take another breath, let it out, and then keep going, breathing in and out, in and out. Start with ten piston breaths, and as the exercise becomes easier, increase the number to twenty, then forty, then sixty, up to a hundred breaths.

EXERCISE 3

Lie on the floor on your back and stretch your arms out by your sides, left palm facing up and right palm facing down. Cross one leg over the other and shift your weight to the opposite side of your body. Let the leg come to rest where you feel most comfortable without bringing the knee up toward the head. Lie still in this position for five minutes. Repeat the exercise using the opposite leg.

EXERCISE 4

This move is excellent for those with a stiff neck. Place your hands behind your head and, keeping your head absolutely straight, apply pressure simultaneously from the head to the hands and the hands to the head. Now push the head forward with the hands and use the head to resist that push. This move stretches the muscles in the neck area, freeing circulation and stimulating the brain. Do this move five times, holding the stretch for a few seconds each time.

EXERCISE 5

This stretch maintains pliability in the lower back. Sit upright in a chair with your thighs parallel to and the lower part of your leg perpendicular to the floor. Bend over, placing your elbows on the inside of your knees, then tuck your fingers under the arch of each foot while placing your thumb over the top of the foot. Let your spine stretch fully in this position. Maintain the pose for five minutes.

EXERCISE 6

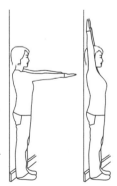

Stand with your back against a wall with your heels, lower back, shoulder blades, and the back of your head touching it. Now raise your arms straight out in front of you, letting your thumbs touch each other. As slowly as possible, raise your arms above your head until you touch the wall. Then lower your arms out and down to your sides. Do this three times, once a day.

Dr. Fulford believed that patients who did these exercises regularly would avoid illness and allow energy to flow freely throughout their bodies. All are beneficial, but Dr. Fulford emphasized that if you were pressed for time, numbers five and six were most important.

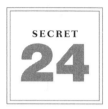

SECRET

24

Vitamin C

SUSAN RENNAU

Back in the late 1960s, most teenagers were listening to
Pink Floyd, the Rolling Stones, and Jimi Hendrix, but not
to their parents. Susan Rennau, now fifty-eight years old,
raised in a New York suburb rife with protests against racism,
marches for Robert F. Kennedy, and vigils for Martin Luther King, was.
"It wasn't cool to like your parents. But unlike many in my generation,
I had a very loving foundation."

Still, there were a few rocky moments in her household, the
worst being the time her parents insisted she attend Catholic school
in nearby New Rochelle. "I made their life miserable until they gave
in and let me attend public school." Her parents were very Catholic;
Susan was "very agnostic." But a bond between mother and daughter
was always present. "What would Mom do?" has been her lifelong
mantra.

Susan attended college in New England, then moved to Utah to ski, figuring she'd stay one season. She never left. She did, however, decide she needed a real job and wound up earning a second bachelor's degree in nursing from the University of Utah. She eventually married, had twin daughters, divorced, and after working at several places, became a nurse coordinator for an outpatient clinic. Today she assists with conscious sedation for gastroenterology patients. "If you are getting a procedure on your digestive tract, I give you the medication that keeps you comfortable."

"THERE'S MORE VITAMIN C in sunflower seeds than anything... and you gotta have a lot of vitamin C to keep going. I eat a lot of them seeds and we use the oil in salads and things like that there. And rose hips tea, I drink that. Got lots of vitamin C in it."

~ENOS SLAUGHTER,
AMERICAN BASEBALL PLAYER

Susan herself was an average patient, becoming sick once or twice a year. Then in 2006, her mother died of lung cancer at age eighty-six. Susan returned home one more time to go through her mother's possessions. Among them she found an enormous container of vitamin C tablets that her mother had taken religiously.

After bringing the jug back to Utah, Susan started taking the pills too. One day, almost a year later, she realized that she hadn't been sick since. So she decided to buy her own jar, and she continues to take vitamin C supplements and remains healthy.

In the spring of 2009, the swine flu swept through the office where she worked. In one week, seven staff members were out sick. Susan remained healthy, despite being exposed to her colleagues *and* their patients.

"It's not only vitamin C. I also have a healthy lifestyle: nutrition, exercise, and temperance. But I've gained an advantage over the cold or sore throat that used to creep up on me once or twice a year. Since I've started taking the C, there have been three or four times I've felt I might be starting to get a sore throat, but then it goes away. And the last four years were very stressful times for me—I decided to divorce, my daughters moved away for college, my mom died. I give credit to my vitamins, the gift my mom provided me. Nice inheritance."

Her daughters don't take C, however. "Maybe in forty years," Susan says, "I'll make sure there's a big jar of vitamin C in the medicine cabinet."

The Facts on Vitamin C

In 2003, the National Institutes of Health designated the Linus Pauling Institute (LPI) as a Center for Excellence in the field of alternative and complementary medicine. (There are only a few such centers in the country.) The institute studies and publishes information on a wide variety of micronutrients, from those in broccoli and garlic to vitamin and mineral supplements. Ongoing LPI seminars mention discussions on the health effects of garlic, broccoli, and vitamins D and E. The star vitamin at the LPI, however—the one that Nobel Prize–winning chemist Linus Pauling himself took daily at more than thirty times the U.S. recommended daily allowance (RDA)—is vitamin C.

Pauling helped to popularize orthomolecular medicine (a term he coined) in 1970, the year he published his hugely influential book *Vitamin C and the Common Cold*. Previously, people thought of vitamin C as something you just had to get enough of, like calcium or iron, to prevent the odd-sounding disease called scurvy.

Because nearly all of us get enough vitamin C in our diet, avoiding scurvy isn't the focus of its modern proponents. Rather, Pauling and vitamin C advocates make two major claims. First, they recommend a daily megadose of vitamin C for optimal health. Second, they maintain that a megadose at the onset of infection helps limit the intensity of illness. For a mild cold, vitamin-C proponent Robert F. Cathcart, MD, recommends taking 30 to 60 grams every twenty-four hours—that's the equivalent of what you'd ingest by eating more than seven hundred oranges in a single day.

And though the vitamin's benefits are most often linked to fighting the common cold, proponents like Cathcart and Pauling recommend

C VERSUS D

◆

When it comes to colds, vitamin C hogs the spotlight. But a new study of almost twenty thousand people suggests a role for vitamin D in preventing colds, too: Those with low levels of the nutrient were more likely to catch one than those with an adequate amount of it. According to research published in *Archives of Internal Medicine*, people with the greatest vitamin D deficiency were 36 percent more likely to suffer respiratory infections than those with the highest levels.

Since many studies have shown that the majority of people living north of the 40th degree of latitude are deficient in vitamin D, a supplement makes sense. Until recently, 1,000 IUs was considered sufficient, but some experts are now calling for a higher dosage, up to 2,000 IUs or even more.

On the other hand, if you live in a climate where sunshine is plentiful, a twenty-minute walk in the sun several times a week will probably allow the body to manufacture enough vitamin D. Unlike other vitamins, vitamin D doesn't have to be obtained through food; exposure to sunlight is the best source.

Few foods offer quantities of vitamin D, but those that do include fatty fishes, such as salmon and mackerel, eggs, and fortified milk and cereal products. One excellent source is a spoonful of pure (not refined) cod liver oil—your grandmother knew best after all.

megadosages for diseases ranging from infections to cardiovascular disease to cancer. Cathcart's system pegs the vitamin C dose necessary to fight mononucleosis at 200 grams or more per twenty-four-hour period.

Why vitamin C?

Vitamin C acts as a catalyst in the body, facilitating and inducing many necessary chemical reactions. It also helps detoxify the natural waste products of cellular metabolism and behaves as an antioxidant. As such, vitamin C acts like a foster home for wayward electrons (free radicals) jettisoned during routine molecular activity. Without antioxidants, these electrons would otherwise float freely about your cells, triggering confusion by trying to attach themselves to nearby molecules. Vitamin C scoops them up and adds them to its own molecule, safely harboring them.

As a 2003 study in the *Journal of the American College of Nutrition* explains, "Vitamin C in humans must be ingested for survival. Vitamin C is an electron donor, and this accounts for all its known functions." Beyond mere survival, the same study suggests it's possible that antioxidants such as vitamin C help prevent "human diseases like atherosclerosis and cancer [that] might occur in part from oxidant damage to tissues." But the study stops short of prescribing vitamin C to ward off cancer. It acknowledges that "diets rich in fruits and vegetables are associated with lower risk of cardiovascular disease and cancer. It is not known whether vitamin C contributes to those benefits."

In other words, it may be the orange itself, and not the vitamin C, that's beneficial. Eating fruits and vegetables high in vitamin C, like oranges and broccoli, is unquestionably good for you. What isn't yet clear is whether supplemental vitamin C—taken as a pill, via syringe, or otherwise—is similarly effective.

Several recent studies of vitamin C suggest it may be. In 2008, universities in England and Portugal showed that doses of the vitamin can repair the body at a submolecular level. And a 2009 study at the University of California, Berkeley found a connection between supplemental doses of vitamin C and a substance called C-reactive protein (CRP), which is found in higher-than-normal levels in people at risk for heart disease. Studies have shown that two months of vitamin C megadosage reduced CRP levels in people whose levels were elevated.

Such reports indicate that taking vitamin C supplements is probably important for maintaining health, and they support the claim that daily doses of vitamin C reduce the risk of contracting a serious ailment.

But what about the second claim—its purported qualities as a quick cure for the common cold? The data there are less supportive.

In 2001, an Australian team undertook the gold standard of clinical trials, performing a double-blind, randomized, long-term study on

SCURVY

◆

Vitamin C is in an unusual case in which a compound is named after the disease it cures. The chemical name for vitamin C, ascorbic acid, comes from the Latin word for scurvy, *scorbutus*. Scurvy is caused by vitamin C deficiency, which, if untreated, leads to the formation of spots on the skin (mostly the legs), spongy gums, bleeding from mucous membranes, and loss of teeth. In an advanced stage, it can be fatal.

The fact that scurvy could be prevented by eating citrus fruit was first proven scientifically by a doctor in the British Royal Navy in the eighteenth century (although the relationship had been suspected for eons), and in 1795 the English started giving their sailors lime juice, which is how they came to be known as Limeys. However, British ships often stored containers of sauerkraut (fermented cabbage) as well, due to its ability to keep without refrigeration. Captain James Cook once ordered 25,000 pounds of kraut to outfit a two-ship voyage. If the tradition had held, Limeys would have been known as Krauts, which would have made World War I confusing.

vitamin C and colds. For eighteen months, four hundred adults were instructed to take megadoses of vitamin C supplements at the first sign of a cold and to continue taking it for two days. The result? Inconclusive.

And in 2007, three Finnish scientists took the investigation further, performing a metastudy of research on vitamin C and colds. Their report states bluntly: In "ordinary people," vitamin C does not prevent colds, although it might shorten their duration. By ordinary people, the scientists meant anyone who was not a skier, soldier, or marathon runner, because the data on these people did show a clear but inexplicable link between supplemental vitamin C and cold prevention.

Vitamin C's ability to prevent a cold may be in question, and even Pauling admitted that it may not be a miraculous substance on its own, but as a component of nature's vitamin C delivery devices—from fruits like oranges to vegetables like broccoli—it is a vital component of miraculous foods.

Share in the Secret

As noted, few people have to worry about getting the National Institutes of Health's RDA of vitamin C: 60 milligrams, the amount found in a single orange or half a glass of orange juice. Nearly everyone in America is meeting that standard, as so many of our foods are fortified with vitamins and minerals, including vitamin C. For example, a bowl of cereal with skim milk contains anywhere from one fourth to one third of the recommended daily dose. Other surprising high sources of vitamin C include potatoes, garlic, asparagus, and peppers.

As with all nutrients, natural and whole foods are more healthful sources than their processed counterparts. Better a potato than a potato chip; better an orange than its juice. And the fresher, the better. The vitamin C found in an apple—20 to 30 milligrams—may lose most or all of its potency after three months of refrigerated storage.

As easy as it may be to get 60 milligrams of vitamin C in your diet, it's important to do so daily. Vitamin C is water soluble, meaning that it is flushed out of the body when we urinate. The body can't store it even if you ingest a surplus. However, the Linus Pauling Institute believes that the RDA for vitamin C is far too low, recommending megadoses of hundreds, thousands, and perhaps tens of thousands of milligrams per day. To obtain that much vitamin C, you have to take supplements.

The most common forms of vitamin C supplement are a stand-alone pill or part of a multivitamin. One vitamin C pill can contain as much as 1,000 milligrams, or sixteen times the RDA. In contrast, most multivitamins contain less, although they typically offer at least 100 percent of the RDA for vitamin C plus a dozen or more vitamins and minerals.

Whether or not the body can absorb nutrients from a pill as effectively as from whole foods is still uncertain. Some doctors suggest that only a few select nutrients can be well absorbed from a pill; others doubt that any can. To be sure, skip the pill and focus on food sources.

ZINC

Zinc is an essential trace element— plants and animals require it to survive. In humans, zinc shows up in roughly one hundred enzymes that keep our bodies functioning. If we don't get enough, our wounds don't heal as quickly, we lose our ability to taste, and our immune systems suffer. In extreme cases, common in less developed countries, people suffer from loss of appetite, skin lesions, stunted growth, and diarrhea.

In the last two decades, however, zinc is best known for vying with vitamin C for the title of best cure-all for colds.

Still, although hundreds of studies have been published examining the power of zinc to bolster the immune system against colds, definitive conclusions haven't been reached. A 2000 study of five hundred people reported a "modest" benefit, while a 2007 analysis of fourteen previous studies concluded that the effectiveness of zinc lozenges "has yet to be established."

However, once you have the cold, zinc may shorten its duration. In a famous 1990s Cleveland Clinic study, a hundred patients received zinc gluconate lozenges within twenty-four hours of contracting a cold, sucking on them every two hours while awake until all cold symptoms had gone away. The results: a significantly shorter duration of symptoms (4.4 days versus 7.6 days) in patients taking the zinc lozenges compared to those given a placebo.

Murking up the issue is the revelation that after these data were compiled but before the study was published, at least one of the researchers bought stock in a company selling zinc lozenges; that stock rose substantially when the study results went public.

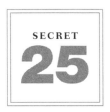

Yoga

FELICE RHIANNON

Felice Rhiannon has always been, by her own description, peripatetic. She has lived all over the world: Taiwan, California, Massachusetts, and currently London. More than where she has lived, she has been colored by the times, particularly by the spirituality that pervaded the 1960s. Felice's interest in being a "spiritual hippie" did not endear her to her mother, who found it incomprehensible; as a result, their relationship suffered.

Nonetheless, sixty-three-year-old Felice pursued her quest, which led her, in her forties, to take a yoga class. When she arrived at the studio, she realized she was the oldest student, and that awkward moment led to an epiphany: She'd bring yoga to people who, like her, thought they were too old for it. Today she's a full-time teacher of the discipline to students who might otherwise feel intimidated or simply uncomfortable in a conventional yoga class. Felice's classes are taught at a slower pace, with carefully articulated instructions, extra rest time, and an emphasis on the less physically difficult poses.

Felice credits yoga for the fact that she herself has no ailments. Her only serious illness came when she lived in Southern California: hemolytic anemia, a genetic blood disorder characterized by a lack of red blood cells. She undertook treatment and has recovered, thanks to her otherwise healthy body. Except for that episode, when flus and colds swept through Los Angeles like the Santa Ana winds, she rarely succumbed—because, she says, of the relaxed, meditative state yoga induces.

"Traditionally, the yoga poses were taught to prepare the body for meditation. What we now call yoga really developed in the last hundred years. Previously, practicing yoga meant you meditated."

After all, in order to sit comfortably in a meditation pose, "No matter what your age," she says, "you need a body that can support your meditation, that won't distract you mentally from your practice by forcing you to focus on aches and pains. You want your mind to focus on exactly what's happening in that moment, not the shopping list, how cute you look in Spandex, or the hunk on the mat next to you."

It was yoga that helped Felice deal with her most recent crisis—her mother's death. Despite their lifelong differences, Felice helped care for her ninety-six year-old mother during her last eight years, on both a practical and intimate level. She oversaw her treatment and sat by her side as she slid downhill, rearranging her mother's body when she was uncomfortable, giving her medications, helping however she could. During this difficult period, Felice calmed herself with yoga and meditation. "If not for my spiritual practice, I could not have done what I did, and certainly not with inner peace."

The Facts on Yoga

Two generations ago, yoga was a mysterious Eastern practice few Americans knew much about. Today it's so common that airport buses in cities from Cleveland to Houston offer free onboard yoga to help relax harried passengers. Fifteen million Americans now say they include some form of yoga in their fitness regimen, and about 75 percent of all American health clubs offer yoga classes.

> "EVERY HUMAN BEING *is the author of his own health or disease."* ~BUDDHA

But long before there were airline delays and fancy gyms on every corner, there was yoga—the pretzel-twisting system of meditative exercise that's designed to enhance overall well-being. The term, which comes from a Sanskrit word meaning "to yoke or join together," refers to the unity of body, mind, and spirit achieved in a successful yoga practice.

Because the technique was handed down orally from teachers to students, yoga's precise beginnings are unknown, but it's thought to have originated more than five thousand years ago in northern India. The *Yoga Sutras,* one of the earliest texts on yoga (it dates from around the year A.D. 1), attempts to organize its previously diverse practices into one system based on eight doctrines, or "limbs." The third, fourth, and fifth of these limbs evolved into modern Western yoga: *asana,* or physical exercises, *pranayama,* or breathing techniques, and *pratyahara,* or meditation (literally, "recovering").

Yoga entered American consciousness in the late nineteenth century, when a master named Swami Vivekananda popularized it in Western nations. However, sun salutations and lotus poses remained curiosities until the 1960s when Eastern spirituality came into vogue, particularly among the young. Suddenly yoga classes were being taught at shopping malls and YMCAs.

Today more than a hundred types of yoga are practiced. Braver souls try power yoga, which does not pause between poses, or Bikram yoga, pioneered by the Olympic gold medal weight lifter Bikram Choudhury, which takes place in rooms heated to a minimum of 105°F. In the United States, the most widely practiced type is the slow and gentle hatha yoga, in which the instructor takes students through a series of poses while helping them become aware of and change their breathing and thought patterns.

THE DOWNSIDE OF YOGA

◆

Like many others, I've tried yoga on and off throughout most of my life. It's both relaxing and strenuous, and when it works, every part of your being, from your brain to your feet, achieves a calm peace.

When it works. Unfortunately, there are more people who want to teach yoga than people who can teach it well. Yoga is neither a game nor a dance step—it's a serious discipline that asks the body to enter positions unfamiliar to Westerners, and which can be painful if done improperly.

The last time I tried yoga was a beginner's class at a well-known spiritual and wellness center. According to the catalog, the teacher was an experienced professional with an outstanding résumé. It turned out that her enthusiasm outweighed her judgment. She pressed the class far too hard. Despite my protests, the teacher insisted I could stretch my back further. I resisted. She pushed. I protested. She insisted. I surrendered. My back snapped. It was the only time in my life I've ever felt real back pain, and it took many sessions with a skilled acupuncturist to recover.

The NIH considers yoga a form of "complementary and alternative medicine," and physicians sometimes recommend it as an adjunct to conventional treatments for a range of chronic conditions, including asthma, back pain, and arthritis. In general, yoga helps the body by:

- *Triggering and enhancing the immune system.* Practitioners claim yoga's body/breath/mind exercises strengthen and balance the immune system, stimulating it to more effectively destroy invading microbes.

- *Relieving stress.* Stress lowers resistance to disease because it reduces the ability of the body to produce disease-fighting immune cells. Yoga stimulates the parasympathetic nervous system (the opposite of our body's fight-or-flight response, which relies on the sympathetic nervous system) by decreasing

191

hormones produced by the adrenal gland in reaction to perceived threats and increasing the body's feel-good hormones.

- *Massaging the organs.* The compression of organs resulting from certain yoga poses resembles the pressure applied during other alternative treatments, such as massage, which stimulate the glands involved in immune-system response. Different yoga poses affect different organs and body systems. For example, the cobra and the bridge, which open the chest and allow deep breathing, stimulate the thymus, while the plow and the downward dog increase lymphatic system function, producing more immune cells to defend against germs. There are even specific poses used to target specific ailments, from high blood pressure to the common cold.

Ongoing research into yoga's ability to treat a variety of conditions, from diabetes to dementia, seems to support such claims. Studies published in a wide variety of medical journals indicate that yoga can lower blood pressure, thus improving circulation and cardiovascular health, lower pulse and respiration rate, improve gastrointestinal function, lower blood glucose, increase the supply of red blood cells, soothe depression and anxiety, and more.

The connection between yoga and heart disease has been particularly well researched. In 1990, as reported in *Dr. Dean Ornish's Program for Reversing Heart Disease* (a book based on a study that focused on diet and exercise instead of drugs and surgery), yoga was found to decrease participants' cholesterol and triglycerides. And in 2007, a study published in the journal *Diabetes Research and Clinical Practice* found that yoga could reverse several heart disease risk factors, including obesity, high blood pressure, and high blood sugar. Participants who practiced yoga also developed higher levels of HDL (healthy) cholesterol.

All that said, risks are involved—especially for beginners or those with certain health problems such as spinal disc disease, glaucoma, or osteoporosis. No studies show that yoga is detrimental to your health if done properly, but the stretches attained can cause as much damage

MEDITATION AND HEART DISEASE

◆

According to a report in the *AAAS News*, the journal of the American Association for the Advancement of Science, a 2009 clinical trial found that meditation cuts the risk of heart attack, stroke, and death by nearly 50 percent in patients with existing coronary heart disease. The report noted that this finding means that meditation is as effective as any of the standard prescription drugs on the market for treating cardiac ailments.

This particular study examined transcendental meditation, the kind introduced to the world in 1955 by Maharishi Mahesh Yogi and made famous by his students, the Beatles. The study found that patients who meditated in addition to taking standard treatment experienced 47 percent fewer heart attacks, strokes, and deaths compared with the control group. In comparison, statin drugs lessened the risk by 30 to 40 percent relative to existing treatments. Common blood-pressure drugs reduced these outcomes by only 25 to 30 percent.

Here as elsewhere, when judging the value of such studies, it's a good idea to look at who's behind them. The study above was completed with a $2.3 million grant from the NIH and the National Heart, Lung and Blood Institute and was conducted by the Medical College of Wisconsin along with the Maharishi University in Iowa, the last of which probably had a stake in the outcome. This doesn't negate the findings by any means, but researching who underwrote and performed a study can provide valuable perspective with which to weigh the evidence.

as much more vigorous exercise. Even seemingly simple postures can present serious risks for some people: For example, the Lotus position puts pressure on weak hip-flexor muscles.

According to a recent *Time* magazine article, medical professionals regularly treat patients with yoga-related injuries. In fact, between 2004 and 2007, the Consumer Product Safety Commission reported some thirteen thousand Americans were treated for such injuries.

Keep in mind that yoga was created to help people understand their bodies and themselves, improving their entire lives rather than treating symptoms of illnesses. As the great yoga teacher B.K.S. Iyengar once said: "Yoga teaches us to cure what need not be endured and endure what cannot be cured."

Share in the Secret

Before starting a yoga practice, consult with your doctor to determine if it may exacerbate any preexisting medical conditions.

Once you're ready, check the Internet, fliers at the gym, health food stores—you'll find that classes in a variety of yoga styles and experience levels are offered in many locales, including most health clubs, specialized yoga studios, and continuing education classes. But before you enroll, make sure your class is run by a qualified (trained and experienced) teacher. There is no standard certification to teach yoga, but the American Yoga Association (AYA) offers suggestions for finding an instructor on their website. Once you find him or her, follow the NIH recommendation: Set up a time to talk and ask about the class's physical demands.

You can also learn and do yoga at home in front of your television using one of the many professional yoga videos available. The AYA offers a *Basic Yoga* DVD and books such as *The American Yoga Association's Beginner's Manual*.

Whichever route you choose, you'll need some comfortable clothing. You can buy special yoga outfits, but any old sweats and a close-fitting T-shirt will do as well. (You can skip the shoes: Yoga is usually performed barefoot.) You'll also need a slender and sticky yoga mat (usually available free at classes or sold at athletic or yoga stores, or online from outlets like Gaiam.com).

Be aware that not all teachers are good ones. Trust your body. If you sense you're pushing it too hard, don't be afraid to stop. You know your body better than anyone else.

Afterword

———————◆———————

Twenty-five different people with twenty-five different health secrets. From bathing in cold H_2O to dowsing in bottled H_2O_2, from downing dirt to doing the downward dog. Secrets from nurses and doctors, firefighters and comedians, agents and politicians. All the people included believe their secret is the reason for their good health. All of them feel very confident. All of them are (or were, during their lifetimes) very healthy.

Still, it quickly became clear to me that these people have conflicting ideas on what helps them stay well. Rip Esselstyn avoids the dairy-based yogurts Tony Japour consumes. Sasha Lodi and Helen Klein don't see eye to eye on exercise. Only Nate Halsey jumps into cold showers. Nobody else avoids people's germs like Rachel Hill does. Most people enjoy garlic, but only Susan Seideman Brown consumes it so systematically.

Given that my quest for these secrets was initiated, in part, to avoid catching colds, it seemed reasonable to adopt as many of these secrets as made sense. The good news is that most of them are easy to add to a daily routine; some of them were already part of mine. For instance when I co-wrote Rip's book, *The Engine 2 Diet,* his unrepressed enthusiasm for a plant-based diet made me want to join in, and I became a member of his Engine 2 pilot study. The results of my lipid tests were impressive enough that eating only plants has been part of my life for several years.

I've been performing many of Dr. Fulford's exercises since ghostwriting his book, *Dr. Fulford's Touch of Life.* Every morning I do the two he told me were most important: sitting in a chair and lengthening the spine, then leaning against a wall and raising the arms to stretch in the opposite direction. These exercises were designed to strengthen the back muscles as well as to enhance overall health, and on that front, back pain has yet to appear in my life (except for that one excruciating yoga ache).

Napping is already integrated into my daily routine, but in the past I ascribed this habit to lethargy. Now I have permission to think the daily snooze is evidence that I'm taking good care of myself. Every day, sometime between 1 and 3 P.M. (the times recommended by Sarnoff's daughter, nap expert Sara Mednick), I sleep—not for as long as she recommends, but for at least fifteen minutes.

Because these secrets alone hadn't been enough to keep me healthy, I added more, assuming that each individual has different needs, and that in my case, a variety of secrets was necessary to stay well. Everyone's system is unique. Whereas for some, one secret may suffice, for others, it may take many. Perhaps some may need all of them.

I also noticed that even though some of the ideas clash with one another, the people interviewed, even if they prefer one secret over all others, don't live in a vacuum. Many exercise aerobically and anaerobically, take vitamin and mineral supplements, eat less than most people, and so on. In other words, they all make an effort to live a healthy, well-balanced life.

For me, the toughest of my new habits is eating raw garlic, which I took up after talking with Susan Brown: I don't do it often, but whenever a cold feels imminent, I chomp on a clove. Some people like the taste; I find the garlic literally difficult to swallow. Still, more than any other of the secrets, my gut tells me it's working on whatever attackers are invading my body.

Due to my plant-based diet, chicken soup and dairy-based yogurt are off-limits, although I do eat soy yogurt with live probiotic cultures now and then.

After hearing Barbara Pritzkat praise the powers of brewer's yeast, I decided to mix a tablespoon of it into my morning health concoction. Unlike the garlic, the taste of the brewer's yeast doesn't bother me, although that might be due to the fact that the rest of the mix contains pomegranate, orange, and cranberry juices, along with a fizzy powder product called Emergen-C, a heaping scoop of Green Vibrance (a nutritional supplement that, says the label, supports "the 4 Foundations of Health: Nutrition, Digestion, Circulation, & Immunity"), and a half teaspoon of flaxseed oil.

The Emergen-C is replete with vitamin C, a nutrient that, thanks to Susan Rennau's recommendation, I now ingest a great deal more of. Coincidentally, when I was an undergraduate at Stanford in the early 1970s, I participated in Dr. Linus Pauling's original vitamin C experiments, ingesting enormous amounts of it. It gave me diarrhea, so I dropped out of the study. Today I take much less, and my system responds much better.

Although I'm not much of a cook, I have added more herbs to my diet (without adding excess salt). And speaking of food, caloric reduction wasn't for me, because I already eat less than most people and don't feel like cutting back any further. Although calorie consumption is primarily a health issue, to some degree it is also a psychological one. For many, food is as much about nurturance as nutrition; they turn to it for comfort. The majority of such people were raised in families where meals played a vital role, and food remains a metaphor for security, relationships, or some other deep significance. However, I grew up in a household where food was of minimal importance. No one cooked it well, no one enjoyed it much, and everyone left the dinner table as quickly as possible. When I feel anxious or unhappy, I turn away from food. My weight hasn't changed much since college.

No matter how much I tried, though, some of these secrets simply didn't take. I attempted jumping into a cold shower, but couldn't acclimate to the idea of facing freezing water in the morning—or any other time, for that matter. Even with Nate Halsey's enthusiastic coaching, being drenched in cold water felt painful. Similarly, I still feel compelled to clean my fruit pretty scrupulously, even though Patricia Burke has explained that that may not be necessary. The habit is too firmly ingrained.

Exercise has always been part of my life, but everyone has his or her own preferences. Even though I'm about the same age as Helen Klein when she took up running, I get bored too easily going long distances. However, my three-times-a-week gym routine does include aerobic exercise as well as weight lifting. So the old regime will suffice for now.

After talking to pH advocate Tom Appell, I bought litmus paper and tested my urine every day for a week, but perhaps because my diet already consists of so many fruits and vegetables, my pH balance was healthy. And peeing on the paper felt awkward. Several times I missed. I tried dunking my head in hydrogen peroxide as well, and although I never missed, I never felt comfortable either, so when the bottle was empty, it wasn't replaced.

Living in Manhattan makes it impossible to avoid the constant sneezing, coughing, and nose blowing of strangers. But washing my hands after this exposure has now become routine. It hadn't occurred to me before to wash them unless they were dirty; now I do it preventively.

Being a city-dweller has also made it possible to make many friends, but unlike Sydney Kling, I haven't cataloged them. It's hard to argue that a social support system isn't a healthy thing; it just never occurred to me that each friend is a potential ally in the fight against illness. This makes my address book a different form of pharmacy.

Finally, although Susan Smith Jones is a passionate advocate for stresslessness, it's nearly impossible to write for a living and remain stress-free. I'm working on her advice points, but I can't pretend that anxiety didn't attack many times when I turned on the computer and this book appeared onscreen. It could have been worse: Watch Jack Nicholson as Jack Torrance in *The Shining*—that's what stress can ultimately do to a writer.

◆

The best part of all these remedies is that in the time it's taken to research and publish this book, my health has unquestionably improved. I still may feel a cold coming on now and then—but that's about it. At no point have I come down with the raging sore throat and red, runny nose of years past. The reason for that may have as much to do with my new belief system as anything else: I truly believe that the combination of secrets I've chosen is working for me.

And that is the one commonality of these secrets. People may take cold showers, drink warm soup, or eat hot spices, but in each case, the person who has shared the secret firmly believes that it is why he or she stays well. This is why, to some degree, everyone in the book agrees with one theory—Gail Evans's attitude about attitude.

Rationally, that may not make much sense. But little in health research does. For nearly every study that claims to prove point A, another study refutes it with point B. Ideas popular in one decade become passé in the next. In the 1960s, doctors considered many of the medical practices of the 1910s somewhat barbaric; today the same is true of some from the 1960s. For instance, consider "completely safe" barbiturates, the overuse of electroshock therapy, or prescription drugs such as Halcion that were considered free of all side effects and yet drove some people into a spiraling depression—as told in author William Styron's frightening account of his own experience, *Darkness Visible*.

All we know for sure about the year 2050 is that its doctors will ridicule some of today's prevailing wisdom.

So much conflicting information, and so many treatments falling in and out of fashion—and yet one theory that's been around since Hippocrates is the belief in a mind-body connection. The way we think about our health may be as important as any other aspect in determining how well we are. Still, modern medical science doesn't understand this role of attitude on health, and plenty of well-documented, double-blind, randomized controlled studies dispute its importance. In fact, until recently, Western medicine was reluctant even to admit that the connection exists. It could be that discussing the two constitutes a tautology; the mind and body may be so connected that you might as well be discussing a pancreas-body connection.

That also may explain why the placebo effect is one of the most powerful and least understood concepts in medicine. A placebo (Latin for "I will please") is an inert pill that seemingly has no real medicinal benefit—and yet often has the same effect as the actual medicine for which it is substituted. Many doctors who have given patients placebos instead of medicine have seen those patients' conditions improve— and many doctors now routinely use placebos in place of prescription drugs. A 2004 study of Israeli physicians reported in the *British Medical Journal* found that as many as 60 percent of them had given placebos to their patients—generally to keep them from taking powerful drugs they didn't need; the figure was 40 percent in a study of Danish doctors. In a 2007 survey of doctors in the Chicago area, 47 percent admitted to using some form of a placebo treatment with their patients. (Controlled studies have been undertaken to investigate this phenomenon, but the results have been inconclusive; the NIH is currently funding several such inquiries.)

It has also been shown numerous times that the more faith a patient has in the remedy he or she is given to combat illness, the more likely it is that the chosen remedy will work. But not only do scientists fail to understand why it's true; they also can't say why it's true for some people and not others. And what of the studies that have shown that the more a patient believes in a doctor's ability to understand him or her and the illness, the more likely it is that the doctor's treatments will work? Why is that so—and why doesn't the phenomenon work for everyone? Again, no one knows.

This does not mean that the twenty-five remedies offered in this book are simply placebos, but perhaps without belief, the remedies might not be quite as effective, which is why the connotation of the word placebo is changing in the twenty-first century: Whereas it once implied something relatively worthless, it's now being investigated as a powerful and real medical device, one that may unlock an entirely new paradigm for medical care. The study of the placebo effect has even led to the examination of its opposite—the *nocebo* (Latin for "I will harm") effect, which occurs when the patient has an unduly negative attitude toward whatever remedy he or she is being offered, invalidating its efficacy. Science is just beginning to work on this one (the word was coined less than fifty years ago). If it holds up, it's more proof that the power resides in the mixture of mind and medication.

Taking care of oneself involves many personal beliefs, however, and my own is that my health will improve as I implement as many of these secrets as make sense to me. Why not believe this? Think of Pascal's wager. The seventeenth-century French philosopher Blaise Pascal asserted that God's existence cannot be proven using reason but that it makes reasonable sense to bet that God exists. Put very simply, if you live your life believing that God exists, you have nothing to lose and everything to gain (you'll go to heaven). If you're wrong, however, you'll have lost nothing. But if you bet that God *doesn't* exist, and you're right, you'll gain nothing, because when you die, it's all over. And if you were wrong, then you really lose, because you'll be consigned to hell for eternity.

I've decided to make an earthly form of Pascal's wager with my health. I choose to believe I've found the correct combination of secrets that will keep me healthy. I have everything to gain from believing it (assuming attitude really does hold sway) and nothing to lose (except perhaps a bad taste in my mouth left by raw garlic). So I intend to keep believing.

Unless for some reason I start getting sick again—in which case my belief system will fly out the window, and I'll need to seek out still more healthy people. (I did make the same kind of bet when I was six concerning the existence of Santa Claus. That one didn't work out so well.) And that means that the publication of this book doesn't end the search for health secrets. If you have a different one that you'd like to share (or an opinion of the ones I've described), please visit www.secretsofpeople.com and post your experiences.

◆

B esides belief, there is something else that everyone in the book shares: consistency. These aren't people who sometimes take a cold shower or occasionally eat probiotics or run now and then. Their secrets are woven into the fabric of their daily routine.

That's the secret to any secret—doing it. Belief is the underlying attitude, but without the practice, nothing is accomplished. If you decide that you want to make one of these secrets your own, take that decision seriously. Don't try it now and then, or when you remember, or only when you feel ill. Whatever you decide to do, do it, and do it as regularly as possible.

Maintaining this consistency means choosing the secrets that make sense for you and your lifestyle. If you enjoy exercising with others but hate the gym, give yoga a try. If solitary workouts are more to your liking, running is the way to go. If you don't have the time or just dislike working out, the diet-based secrets will be easier to stomach.

Once you try one, stick with it—at least long enough to determine if it's right for you. I knew quickly that cold showers, no matter how healthy they might be, were never going to be a part of my life. Eating a plant-based diet took some time to adjust to; at first it required serious effort, but now it's a snap, and I seldom stray from it. Adding brewer's yeast to my morning drink was as easy as buying it at the health food store and storing it next to the drink's other ingredients.

Pick a secret that makes sense for you and your lifestyle. Pick one that appeals to your strength. Pick one that your friends and family will support. Don't be upset if you try one and it doesn't work. Try another.

Good health results from good healthy habits. No matter which secret becomes yours, make it a part of your life.

Acknowledgments

Many of the people in this book are friends, and some have become friends once I interviewed them, so if Sydney Kling is correct about social networks, I should be that much healthier. I am especially grateful to those who took time from their busy days to talk: Tom Appell, Susan Seideman Brown, Patricia Burke, Phil Damon, Rip Esselstyn, Gail Evans, Ricardo Osorno Fallas, Nate Halsey, Rachel Hill, Tony Japour, Susan Smith Jones, John Joseph, Helen Klein, Sydney Kling, Sasha Lodi, Sarnoff Mednick, Barbara Pritzkat, Susan Rennau, Felice Rhiannon, and Bill Thompson.

The following people were very helpful and deserve thanks: Doug Abrams, Al and Sheryl Attanasio, David Auchincloss, Diana Baroni, Scott Beale, Jess Brallier, Sally Chabert, Pip Coburn, John Coyne, Mark and Monica Cravotta, Susie Crile, Arturo Cruz Jr., Mark Davis, Laurie Dolphin, Jon Doyle, Felice Dunas, Roger Emert, Alan Emtage, Ann and

Essy Esselstyn, Zeb Esselstyn, Larry Ford, Russell Gordon, Vicki Gordon, Doug Green, Greg Greene, Duke Greenhill, Nathan Greenlee, Mary Gwynn, Josh Hammer, John Hartmann, Steve Hirshhorn, Dorothea Hover-Kramer, Rick Kellerman, Polly King, Peter Kingham, Jill Kolasinski, Rick Kot, Heidi Krupp, Adam Kushner, Polly Labarre, George Lattimore, Renee Lattimore, Tara Lattimore, Ronna Lichtenberg, Mark Liponis, Arthur Lubow, Sidney Mackenzie, John Marcom, Barbara Marcus, Kathy Matthews, Marc McMorris, Sara Mednick, Sandi Mendelson, Howard Menikoff, Susan Mercandetti, Leslie Mish, Victoria Moran, Mary Murphy, Blake Mycoskie, David Noonan, Becky Okrent, Judith Orloff, Mike Otterman, Jennifer Peters, Carl Pritzkat, Eric Rayman, Donna Redel, Michael Rhodes, Susan Roberts, Robin Rue, Tim Sanders, John Scheidt, Kent Sepkowitz, Stanley Siegel, Glenn Sinclair, Jim Stewart, Mark Sutton, Tony Travostino, Rich Turner, Don Weisberg, Jen White, Bryant Wieneke, Rafe Yglesias, and Jon Zornow.

I am especially grateful to my excellent agent, Richard Pine, because we hatched this book together. Luckily, he didn't want to write it.

At Workman, I owe thanks to Janet Vicario, David Matt, E. Y. Lee, Kevin Davidson, Nathan Lifton, Beth Levy, Barbara Peragine, Julie Primavera, Walter Weintz, Page Edmunds, Beth Wareham, James Wehrle, Joe Ginis, Steven Pace, Jenny Mandel, Jodi Weiss, Michael Rockliff, David Schiller, Andrea Fleck-Nisbet, Justin Nisbet, Kristina Peterson, Sara High, Melissa Broder, Brian Lucas, Peter Workman, Bob Miller, and especially to my editor and friend Suzie Bolotin, who is not only healthy but very, very wise.

I particularly want to thank Isaac Cherem, Mike Terry, and Nick Earhart for their research; Miranda Spencer, an excellent editor and friend; William Callahan, who contributed a great deal to this book; and most of all Tetsuhiko Endo, a good writer and a good surfer, both on the Web and the waves.

Index

A

Acidifying foods, 121.
    See also pH balance
Acidosis, 121–22
Acne, 12
Aerobic exercise, 151, 152, 156
    running, 149–56, 198
Aging process, xii, 15, 84,
    143
AIDS, 141, 142
Alcohol, xiv, 12–13, 14–15, 22, 33, 43,
    44, 146
Alkalizing foods, 121, 123.
    See also pH balance
Allergies:
    to Alliums, 66
    hygiene hypothesis and, 50–54
Alzheimer's disease, 15, 21, 128, 137
Anaerobic exercise, 103–4, 105, 151
    weight lifting, 100–108, 151, 198
Animals, contact with, xii–xiii, 54, 72,
    73
Antibiotics, 66, 75, 90, 142–43, 146
Antioxidants, 15, 37, 66, 88, 89, 90, 91,
    183–84
Aortic dissection, 104–5

Appell, Thomas, 118–20, 198
Apples, xii
Aristotle, 61
Arsenic, xiv, 67
Art, 164–65
Arthritis, xiii, 97, 135, 137
Asclepius, 161
Asthma, 52–53, 170
Atherosclerosis, 66, 184
Athlete's foot, 72, 97
Ayurvedic remedies, 90

B

Back disorders, 137, 170, 177
Bacteria, 72. *See also* Germs
    antibiotics and, 143
    hygiene hypothesis and, 50–53
    probiotics and, 142–48
Baths, detoxifying, 46
Béchamp, Antoine, 120–21
Bed sharing with partner, 112–13
Bedsores, xiii
Beer making, 12, 16
Bee stings, xiii
Biofeedback, 137, 138

Blackburn, Elizabeth H., 84–85
Bladder infections, xii
Bloodletting, xiii, xiv, 73
Blood pressure, xii–xiii, 21, 65, 91, 137, 144. See also High blood pressure
weight training and, 104–5
Blue Zones, 3–9
Bone density, 104, 122, 155
Breast cancer, 59, 82, 84, 104, 153
Brewer's yeast, 10–17, 197
Brown, Susan Seideman, 63–64, 69, 197
Buddha, 190
Buettner, Dan, 5, 8, 9
Burke, Patricia, 48–49, 54, 198
Burns, George, 18–19, 24, 25
B vitamins, 11, 13–14, 16, 89, 130

C

Caffeine, 117
Callahan, Gerald, 53, 54
Caloric reduction, xi–xii, 6, 9, 18–26, 197
Campbell, T. Colin, 129
Cancer, xii, xiv, xv, 5, 6, 15, 45, 59, 65, 82, 84–85, 88, 97, 104, 106, 119, 127, 128, 129, 144, 153, 183, 184
animal products and, 129
positive attitude and, 134–35, 137, 138
Cannon, Walter B., 169
Capsaicin, 93
Cardiovascular disease, 6, 8, 21, 154, 183, 184. See also Heart disease
Carnegie, Dale, 61–62
Cathcart, Robert F., 182–83
Cayenne pepper, 89, 93

Centenarians, 5, 147
Chicken soup, 27–33
Chile peppers, 93
China:
ancient, 102
traditional medicine in, 35, 86–87, 106
Cholesterol, 21, 65, 66, 88, 125, 126–27, 144, 192
Choudhury, Bikram, 190
Christian Science, 158
Chromosomes, 81–82
telomeres at tips of, 83–85
Cinnamon, 90, 93
Cocaine, xiv, xv
Cod liver oil, 183
Coffee, xiii, xiv, 101, 117
Cognitive problems, xii, 59
Alzheimer's disease, 15, 21, 128, 117
Cold, common, xiv, xvii–xviii, 35, 51, 60, 66, 95, 114, 142, 170, 196
beneficial effects of, 175
chicken soup and, 27–33
echinacea and, 92
feeding, 47
having two at once, 31
vitamin C and, 181–82, 184–85
zinc and, 187
Cold showers, 34–38, 198
Colonics, 41
Consistency, 202–3
Cook, James, 185
Copper bracelets, xiii
Cornaro, Luigi, ix–xii, 20
Cortisol, 113–14
Cousins, Norman, 136–37
Cranberry juice, xii
C-reactive protein (CRP), 184

D

Damon, Philip, 39–41
Dannon, 145–46
Darwin, Charles, 82, 128
Davis, Adelle, 10–11, 13, 16, 17
Dehydroepiandrosterone (DHEA), 107
Deoxyribonucleic aid (DNA), 82, 84, 85, 88
Depression, xv, 59, 97, 104, 153, 154, 161, 164, 168, 170, 192, 199
Detoxification, 39–47, 183–84
Diabetes, 8, 21, 33, 50, 83, 105, 116, 121, 127, 153, 170
Diet, 6, 8, 83, 84, 101, 172.
     See also Eating
     caloric reduction and, xi–xii, 6, 9, 18–26, 197
     pH balance and, 118–24
     plant-based, 85, 122–23, 125–32, 196
Diets, fad, 22–23
Dioxins, 43
Dirt:
     eating, 48–54, 130
     playing in, 52
Dogs, xii–xiii, 42–43
Dutch Farmine Study, 83

E

Eating. *See also* Diet
     chicken soup, 27–33
     dirt, 48–54, 130
     garlic, 63–69, 101, 197
     psychological factors and, 197–98
Echinacea, 65, 92
Eczema, 50–53
Eddy, Mary Baker, 158
Edison, Thomas, 20, 112

Egypt, ancient, 12, 14, 35, 65, 102, 161
Endorphins, 137, 139, 154, 172
Enemas, 41, 46
Environmental consciousness, 7
Epigenetics, 83–85
Esselstyn, Caldwell, 128
Esselstyn, Rip, 125–27, 196
Eugenics, 81
Evans, Gail, 133–34, 199
Exercise, 8, 33, 60, 85, 123, 198
     aerobic vs. anaerobic, 151
     health benefits of, 151–55, 172
     lifting weights, 100–108, 151, 198
     running, 149–56, 198
     stretching, 173–79, 196

F

Fad diets, 22–23
Fasting, 41, 45–46
Fat intake, 26, 85, 129
"Feed a cold, starve a fever," 47
Fermentation, 12–13
Fever, xviii, 47, 65, 175
Fight-or-flight response, 44, 57, 169, 170
Fire cupping, 96–97
Fish, xii, 183
Flavonoids, 15
Fletcher, Horace, 22–23
Flu, xviii, 47, 96, 181
Fluid intake, 172
Formaldehyde, 43
Free radicals, 88, 97, 183–84
Freud, Sigmund, xiv
Friends, 55–62, 198
Fulford, Robert, 173–75, 173–79, 196
Full moon, xii
Fungi, 72.
     See also Germs

G

Galen, 151–52, 161

Galton, Sir Francis, 81, 162

Garlic, 63–69, 101, 197

Genetics, 8, 33, 53, 57

    good, 79–85

Germs (pathogens):

    avoiding, 70–78

    hydrogen peroxide and, 95

    hygiene hypothesis and, 50–54, 72

    illnesses caused by (germ theory),

        xviii, 72–77, 120

    living outside human being, 76

Ginger, 89, 93

Ginseng, 87, 89, 91–93

Goddell, Mrs., 27–28

Gold therapy, xiii

Gotu kola, 88–89

Gratitude, attitude of, 172

Greece, ancient, 14, 35, 103,

    151–52, 161

Green tea, 88, 91

H

Halsey, Nate, 34–35, 38, 198

Hand washing, xviii, 54, 71, 72, 73–74,

    76, 77, 78, 198

Hay fever, 50–53

Heart attack, 15, 83, 114, 154, 169, 170,

    193

Heart disease, 6, 14–15, 32, 50, 59,

    82–83, 104, 105, 110–11, 127,

    128, 129, 153, 154, 170, 192, 193

Heavy metals, 42

Hemlock, xiv

Hemorrhoids, 28, 40

Herbal remedies, 86–93

Herbicides, 43

Herbs, in diet, 197

High blood pressure, 29, 32, 44, 84, 88,

    104, 127, 153, 170, 192

Hildegard of Bingen, Saint, 65

Hill, Rachel, 70–72

Hippocrates, 35, 65, 81, 103, 136, 200

Homocysteine, 13–14

Hookworms, 54

Hughes, Howard, 75

Hume, Mick, 170–71

Hydrogen peroxide, 94–99, 198

Hydrotherapy, 35–36, 41

Hygiene hypothesis, 50–54, 72, 130

Hypertension. *See* High blood pressure

I

Immune system, 13, 35, 37, 88, 89, 97,

    106, 126, 129

    exercise and, 153, 155

    friendships and, 59

    hygiene hypothesis and, 50–54, 72

    liquid gold and, xiii

    probiotics and, 144–45, 146

    sleep and, 114

    spirituality and, 162

    stress and, 83, 167, 170

    yoga and, 191

    zinc and, 187

Immunity, 49, 51

Inflammation, 59, 65, 144

    hygiene hypothesis and, 50–53

Insecticides, 43

Interleukin-6, 162

Iyengar, B.K.S., 194

J

Japour, Tony, 141–42

Jones, Susan Smith, 166–68, 172,

    199

Joseph, John, 157–59, 163

K

Klein, Helen, 149–51, 153, 156, 198
Kling, Sydney, 55–57, 198
Kneipp, Sebastian, 36

L

LaLanne, Jack, 152–53
Laughter, 172
Lavender, 117
Leeches, xiii
Leeuwenhoek, Anton Van, 74
Lemongrass, 89, 93
Lerner, Max, 58
Li Ching-yuen, 86–87
Lifting weights, 100–108, 151, 198
Liver, 44, 45, 88, 89
Lodi, Sasha, 100–102, 104
Loneliness, 60
Longevity, 14, 20, 87, 104, 147
  in Blue Zones, 3–9
Lourdes, France, 159–60, 163

M

Maggots, xiii, 96
Mamadou, Moussa, 79–80
Marital bed, 112–13
Mechnikov, Ilya, 143
Meditation, 36, 139, 164, 167, 168, 172, 189, 193
Mednick, Sara, 111, 114–15, 196
Mednick, Sarnoff, 109–11
Mendel, Gregor, 81
Merck Manual, xiv
Mesopotamia, 160
Metabolic syndrome, 105
Methylation, 83
Middle Ages, xiii, 13, 65, 90
Milo of Croton, 103

Mind-body connection, 200
  placebo effect and, 134–35, 136, 200–201
  positive attitude and, 133–40, 199
  spirituality and, 157–65
Moore, Thomas, 164
Morris, Jeremy, 154
Moseley, Bruce, 135
Multiple sclerosis, xiii
Muscle mass, 101, 103, 104
Mutations, 82, 84
Mysophobia, 74–75, 77

N

Napoléon Bonaparte, 7, 112
Napping, 109–17, 196
National Center for Complementary and Alternative Medicine (NCCAM), 66, 98, 144
Natural selection, 82
Nature, connecting with, 164
Nautilus equipment, 103
Neurasthenia, 169
Neuroticism, 168
Nitrates, 43
Nocebo effect, 201
Nose picking, 51

O

Obesity, 6, 7, 15, 20, 22, 33, 60, 82, 192
Oldenburg, Ray, 58
Opiates, xiv–xv
Orgasms, 107
Orloff, Judith, 139–40
Ornish, Dean, 128–29, 192
Orthomolecular medicine, 182
Osorno Fallas, Ricardo, 3–9
Osteoarthritis, xiii, 137
Osteopathy, 176–77

Osteoporosis, 104, 122, 127, 192
Oxytocin, 57

P

Pascal, Blaise, 201
Pasteur, Louis, 13, 65, 74, 120, 143
Patent medicines, xiv–xv, 23
Pauling, Linus, 182–83, 185, 197
Peale, Norman Vincent, 138
pH, meaning of term, 120
pH balance, 118–24, 129, 198
   urine testing and, 123
Phthalates, 42–43
Pine, Richard, 19
Placebo effect, 134–35, 136, 200–201
Plague, 65, 73
Plant-based diet, 85, 122–23,
   125–32, 196
Playing in dirt, 52
Pliny the Elder, 65
Polychlorinated biphenyls (PCBS), 43
Polyphenols, 88
Positive attitude, 133–40, 199
Prayer, 162, 165
Primate diets, 128
Pritzkat, Barbara, 10–11, 197
Probiotics, 141–48
Processed foods, 33, 40, 123
Prostate cancer, 84–85, 106, 129
Protein intake, 26, 129
Protozoa, 72. *See also* Germs
Puerperal fever, xviii
Purple coneflower, 92
Pythagoras, 132

R

Radithor, 98
Rapid eye movement (REM), 115
Reading, spiritual, 165

Religious faith, 157–65
Rennau, Susan, 180–82, 197
Rhiannon, Felice, 188–89
Rhubarb, 89–90, 93
Rome, ancient, 14, 35, 112, 161
Roosevelt, Teddy, 152
Running, 149–56, 198

S

Salt, 32–33
Sanders, Tim, 61–62
Saunas, 46
Scurvy, 182, 185
Seizures, xii
Self-esteem, 57, 106
Selye, Hans, 169
Semmelweis, Ignaz, xviii, 73–74
Sepkowitz, Kent, 76
Sexual intercourse, 81, 106–7
Shintoism, 36
Shoeless running, 155–56
Short-wave sleep (SWS), 115
Showers, cold, 34–38, 198
Sitting for long periods of time, 105
Sleep, 106
   inadequate, 110, 113–14, 172
   napping and, 109–17, 196
   polyphasic, 111, 112
   stages of, 115
Sloan, Richard P., 162–63
Smoking, 23, 60
Snake oil, xv
Sociability, genetics and, 57
Social networks, 7, 9, 55–62, 198
Soft drinks, xv, 6, 10–11
Sour milk, 143–44
Spirituality, 157–65
Stanley, Clark, xv
Staphylococcus, 53, 66

Still, Andrew Taylor, 176
Strachan, David, 50
Strength training, 100–108, 151, 198
Streptococcal diseases, 90, 170
Stress, 37, 58–59, 83–84, 85, 106, 113–14, 139, 146, 168–71
  avoiding, 7, 8, 123, 166–72, 199
  exercise and, 153–54
  friendships and, 57, 58–59
  harmful effects of, 169–71
  immune system and, 83, 167, 170
  pH balance and, 123
  positive effects of, 170–71
  in teens, 171
  yoga and, 191–92
Stretching, 173–79, 196
Stroke, 14, 21, 32, 114, 128, 193
Styron, William, 199
Sumer, ancient, 12, 14, 65, 160
Sweet Potato–Vegetable Lasagna, 131–32
Swine flu, 73, 181

T

Tapeworms, 23
Tea, 88, 91, 101
Telomeres, 83–85
Tesla, Nikola, 74–75
Thompson, Bill, 94–95, 97, 99
Toxics and toxins, 40, 42–43, 44–45
  detoxification and, 39–47, 183–84
Trepanation, xiii
Triglycerides, 21, 65, 192
Tuberculosis, 170
Type A personalities, 169, 170

U

Urine, testing pH balance of, 123
Urine therapy, 97

V

Vaccination, 49, 75
Veganism, 125–32
Vegetarianism, 127, 132
Viruses, 51, 67, 72, 78, 118.
  See also Germs
  hygiene hypothesis and, 50–53
Vitamin A, 89
Vitamin C, 6, 8, 89, 90, 180–86, 197
Vitamin D, xv, 130, 182, 183
Vitamin K, 90, 144
Vivekananda, Swami, 190

W

Washington, George, xiv, 72–73
Water, 6, 120, 123, 172
Weight, 82. *See also* Obesity
  fad diets and, 22–23
  sleep and, 114, 172
Weight lifting, 100–108, 151, 198
Weil, Andrew, 173, 174, 177
White blood cells, 37, 83, 155
William the Conqueror, 22
Wine, 15, 16
Worrying, 168, 171
Wounds, 96, 97, 187

Y

Yeasts, 12
  Brewer's, 10–17, 197
  nutritional, 16–17
Yoga, 35, 46, 188–94
Yogurt, 122, 142, 144, 145–46, 147
Young, Robert O, 122, 123

Z

Zinc, 187
Zoonoses, 73